METABOLIC RESET COOKBOOK FOR SENIORS

Complete Guide for Seniors to Repair Liver & Revitalize Health, Lose Weight, Limitless Energy & Longevity with Delicious Recipes and 28-Day Meal Plan

Andrew H. Steve

About the Author

Andrew H. Steve, a renowned nutrition and health expert, specializes in empowering individuals over 40 to reclaim their health. With a passion for nutrition and a deep understanding of the human body and metabolism, Andrew has successfully guided many to achieve significant weight loss and enhanced well-being.

With over a decade of experience, Andrew's approach is far from one-size-fits-all. He tailors his advice to each individual, focusing on a holistic method that encompasses a balanced diet, mindful eating, and an active lifestyle, rather than just diets and restrictions.

Known for his ability to distill complex dietary concepts into practical, actionable strategies, Andrew is a guiding force in navigating the intricacies of metabolism and wellness. His dedication extends beyond his professional achievements, as he finds joy in outdoor activities, experimenting with new recipes, and engaging in healthy discussions.

If you're over 40 and looking to lose weight, increase energy, or improve your overall well-being, Andrew H. Steve is your ideal mentor. Under his guidance, you're not just adopting a healthy lifestyle; you're embarking on a transformative journey to rediscover your vitality and thrive.

TABLE OF CONTENTS

INTRODUCTION 12

Purpose of the Cookbook 12

Understanding Metabolism in Seniors 14

CHAPTER ONE 17

Metabolism and Aging 17

How Metabolism Changes with Age 17

Common Metabolic Challenges for Seniors 20

CHAPTER TWO 23

Lifestyle Habits for Metabolic Health 23

Incorporating Physical Activity 23

Stress Management and Sleep...26

CHAPTER THREE...30

Essential Nutrients for Seniors..........................30

Vitamins and Minerals Importance 30

Hydration Tips for Metabolic Health 33

BREAKFAST RECIPES 37

Quinoa Breakfast Bowl 37

Greek Yogurt Parfait 38

Spinach and Feta Omelette...39

Chia Seed Pudding with Berries......................................40

Whole-Grain Pancakes with Banana and Walnuts 41

Avocado and Salmon Toast 42

Blueberry and Almond Smoothie Bowl 43

Sweet Potato and Kale Breakfast Hash 44

Oatmeal with Apples and Cinnamon 45

Egg and Vegetable Breakfast Wrap 46

Blueberry Almond Overnight Oats 47

Veggie Egg Muffins 48

Cinnamon Apple Quinoa Porridge 49

Smoked Salmon and Avocado Bagel 50

Quinoa and Berry Breakfast Parfait 50

Banana Walnut Breakfast Smoothie 51

Sweet Potato and Kale Frittata 52

Berry Protein Pancakes 53

Mediterranean Egg Wrap 54

Pumpkin Spice Chia Seed Pudding 55

LUNCH RECIPES **57**

Grilled Chicken Salad with Citrus Vinaigrette 57

Salmon and Quinoa Stuffed Bell Peppers 58

Mushroom and Spinach Quiche 59

Turkey and Vegetable Stir-Fry with Brown Rice 60

Caprese Chicken Wrap 61

Lentil and Vegetable Soup 62

Shrimp and Quinoa Bowl 63

Mediterranean Chickpea Salad 64

Turkey and Veggie Wrap with Hummus 65

Vegetarian Stuffed Bell Peppers 66

Quinoa and Vegetable Stir-Fry 67

Turkey and Lentil Soup 68

Mediterranean Chickpea Wraps 69

Chicken and Avocado Lettuce Wraps 70

Baked Salmon with Lemon Dill Sauce 71

Quinoa and Black Bean Stuffed Peppers 72

Turkey and Vegetable Skewers 73

Eggplant and Chickpea Curry 74

Spinach and Mushroom Omelette 76

Tofu and Vegetable Skillet 77

DINNER RECIPES **79**

Grilled Salmon with Lemon-Dill Sauce 79

Mediterranean Chicken Skewers 80

Quinoa and Vegetable Stuffed Bell Peppers 81

Baked Chicken with Rosemary and Lemon 82

Shrimp and Asparagus Stir-Fry 83

Lentil and Vegetable Curry 84

Turkey and Vegetable Stir-Fry 85

Chickpea and Spinach Stew 86

Vegetable and Tofu Stir-Fry 87

Baked Eggplant Parmesan 89

Lemon Garlic Herb Baked Chicken 90

Lentil and Vegetable Stir-Fry 91

Mediterranean Turkey Burgers 92

Teriyaki Salmon with Stir-Fried Vegetables 93

Cauliflower and Chickpea Curry 94

Balsamic Glazed Chicken with Roasted Vegetables 95

Spaghetti Squash with Turkey Bolognese 97

Seared Tofu with Quinoa and Broccoli 98

Stuffed Bell Peppers with Quinoa and Black Beans 99

Shrimp and Vegetable Skewers 100

SIDE DISHES 102

Quinoa and Vegetable Pilaf 102

Roasted Brussels Sprouts with Balsamic Glaze 103

Garlic and Herb Cauliflower Mash 104

Spinach and Mushroom Salad with Lemon Vinaigrette 105

Lemon Garlic Asparagus 106

Cucumber and Avocado Salad 107

Sweet Potato and Kale Hash 108

Greek Quinoa Salad 109

Butternut Squash and Cranberry Quinoa 110

Grilled Eggplant with Tomato Salsa 111

Quinoa and Black Bean Stuffed Peppers 112

Garlic Roasted Broccoli 113

Cauliflower and Chickpea Tabbouleh 114

Zucchini Noodles with Pesto 115

Roasted Butternut Squash with Sage 116

Asparagus and Tomato Frittata 118

Green Bean Almondine 119

Beet and Orange Salad 120

Lemon Herb Roasted Potatoes 121

Miso Glazed Eggplant 122

SALAD RECIPES 124

Mediterranean Quinoa Salad 124

Spinach and Berry Salad 125

Shrimp and Avocado Salad 126

Grilled Chicken Caesar Salad 127

Caprese Salad with Balsamic Glaze 128

Asian-Inspired Chicken Salad... 129

Tuna and White Bean Salad... 130

Roasted Vegetable Quinoa Salad.. 131

Waldorf Chicken Salad 132

Roasted Beet and Goat Cheese Salad 133

Superfood Kale Salad with Citrus Vinaigrette................................. 134

Salmon and Avocado Caesar Salad 135

Beet and Quinoa Power Salad.. 136

Chickpea and Tomato Summer Salad.. 137

Quinoa and Mango Summer Salad 138

Pomegranate and Walnut Spinach Salad 139

Southwest Black Bean and Corn Salad... 140

Greek Orzo Salad with Feta.. 141

Apple and Walnut Chicken Salad 142

Quinoa and Broccoli Detox Salad.. 143

SOUP RECIPES.. **145**

Quinoa and Vegetable Minestrone Soup 145

Lentil and Spinach Soup 146

Chicken and Wild Rice Soup... 147

Tomato Basil Quinoa Soup.. 148

Butternut Squash and Apple Soup 149

Spinach and White Bean Soup 150

Miso and Mushroom Soup 151

Turmeric and Ginger Carrot Soup 152

Cabbage and White Bean Soup 153

Chicken and Barley Vegetable Soup 154

Sweet Potato and Kale Lentil Soup 156

Cauliflower and Turmeric Soup 157

Artichoke and White Bean Soup 158

Broccoli and Quinoa Chowder 159

Spiced Carrot and Red Lentil Soup 160

Mushroom and Wild Rice Soup 161

Lemon Chickpea and Kale Soup 162

Beet and Quinoa Soup 163

Black Bean and Corn Soup 164

Asparagus and Quinoa Soup 165

SEAFOOD RECIPES.....................................167

Lemon Garlic Baked Salmon 167

Grilled Shrimp Skewers with Herbs 168

Baked Cod with Tomato and Olive Tapenad 169

Citrus Glazed Grilled Swordfish 170

Poached Halibut with Herbed Lemon Sauce 171

Garlic Butter Baked Shrimp 172

Asian-Inspired Grilled Tuna Steaks 173

Mediterranean Baked Haddock 174

Cilantro Lime Grilled Red Snapper 175

Baked Miso Glazed Cod 176

Herb-Crusted Baked Tilapia 177

Coconut-Curry Shrimp Stir-Fry 178

Almond-Crusted Cod with Mango Salsa 179

Teriyaki Glazed Salmon 180

Lemon Herb Baked Scallops 181

Pesto Grilled Trout 182

Baked Crab-Stuffed Avocado 183

Cumin-Spiced Grilled Mahi-Mahi 184

Lemon Dill Baked Oysters 185

Spicy Garlic Grilled Squid 186

28 DAY MEAL PLAN **188**

CONCLUSION **194**

INTRODUCTION

Purpose of the Cookbook

The main goal of the painstakingly created "Metabolic Reset Cookbook for Seniors" is to enable seniors to proactively control and optimize their metabolic health through a thoughtful and nourishing culinary approach. This cookbook aims to alter the culinary scene for the elderly demographic by providing a thorough guidance in a world where aging frequently brings with it metabolic difficulties.

1. **Educational Empowerment:**

   - The cookbook endeavors to educate seniors about the intricate relationship between aging and metabolism. By providing accessible information, it aims to empower them to make informed dietary choices that align with their specific metabolic needs.

2. **Metabolic Health Enhancement:**

   - Focused on rejuvenating metabolic function, the cookbook offers a collection of recipes curated with precision to include nutrient-dense, metabolism-boosting ingredients. Each recipe is designed not only for its palatability but also for its potential to support and enhance metabolic processes.

3. **Promoting Balanced Nutrition:**

   - A key purpose of the cookbook is to guide seniors in constructing well-balanced and nutritionally dense meals.

Through insights on portion control, essential nutrients, and meal planning, the cookbook equips seniors with the tools needed to maintain a healthful diet.

4. **Practical Culinary Solutions:**

   - Acknowledging the diverse lifestyles and preferences of seniors, the cookbook emphasizes practicality in the kitchen. It offers simple yet flavourful recipes, and insights into easy cooking techniques, ensuring that seniors can effortlessly integrate healthy culinary practices into their daily lives.

5. **Tailored to Special Needs:**

   - Recognizing that health needs vary, the cookbook includes chapters dedicated to special dietary considerations. Whether managing diabetes, adhering to a low-sodium diet, or navigating allergen restrictions, seniors will find tailored recipes that suit their unique requirements.

6. **Encouraging Lifestyle Habits:**

   - Beyond the kitchen, the cookbook advocates for a holistic approach to metabolic health. It provides guidance on lifestyle habits, including physical activity, stress management, and adequate sleep, reinforcing the idea that a comprehensive approach is crucial for overall well-being.

7. **Inspiration and Motivation:**

- Featuring success stories from individuals who have experienced positive transformations through the adoption of the cookbook's principles, it serves as a source of inspiration and motivation. These real-life examples underscore the transformative impact that mindful eating can have on metabolic health.

Understanding Metabolism in Seniors

Changes in metabolism are among the many intricate and natural changes that occur in the body as people age. The body's overall biochemical processes, or metabolism, are what determine how nutrients are used, energy is created, and general health is preserved. Customizing dietary and lifestyle practices that support optimal health requires an understanding of the subtleties of metabolism in the elderly.

1. **Metabolic Rate Changes:**

- Aging is associated with a gradual decline in metabolic rate. This reduction is primarily due to a decrease in lean muscle mass and changes in hormonal levels. Understanding this decline is essential for seniors as it impacts daily energy requirements and influences weight management.

2. **Nutrient Absorption and Utilization:**

- Seniors may experience alterations in the absorption and utilization of nutrients. Factors such as changes in digestive enzymes, stomach acid levels, and intestinal function can affect how the body processes and assimilates essential nutrients like vitamins and minerals. This understanding underscores the importance of nutrient-dense dietary choices.

3. **Insulin Sensitivity and Blood Sugar Regulation:**

   - Aging is often associated with decreased insulin sensitivity, potentially leading to challenges in blood sugar regulation. Seniors may be more prone to conditions like insulin resistance or Type 2 diabetes. A nuanced understanding of these metabolic changes is vital for creating meal plans that support stable blood sugar levels.

4. **Muscle Mass Preservation:**

   - Loss of muscle mass, known as sarcopenia, is a common age-related change. Since muscle tissue is metabolically active, its reduction can contribute to a slower metabolism. Strategies to preserve and build muscle through appropriate nutrition and resistance training become crucial elements in supporting metabolic health.

5. **Influence of Hormones:**

   - Hormonal fluctuations, including changes in growth hormone, thyroid hormones, and sex hormones, are part of the aging process. These changes can impact metabolic function. Recognizing the role of hormones in metabolism helps in tailoring dietary recommendations that address specific needs associated with hormonal shifts.

6. **Dietary Protein Requirements:**

   - Adequate protein intake becomes increasingly important for seniors to support muscle maintenance and repair. Understanding the optimal balance of macronutrients, with an emphasis on protein, assists in crafting meals that meet the specific nutritional needs of seniors.

7. **Hydration and Metabolic Function:**

   - Age-related changes in thirst perception and kidney function can contribute to dehydration, affecting metabolic processes. Seniors may need to be more conscious of staying adequately hydrated to support optimal metabolic function.

8. **Adapting to Lifestyle Changes:**

   - Lifestyle factors, including physical activity levels and stress management, significantly influence metabolism. As seniors may experience changes in mobility and daily activities, adapting lifestyle habits becomes integral for supporting metabolic health.

CHAPTER ONE

Metabolism and Aging

How Metabolism Changes with Age

The natural and dynamic process of aging includes many physiological changes, with metabolism being one area that is significantly impacted. As people age, their metabolism, which is the culmination of all biochemical processes in the body, changes. It is essential to comprehend these changes in order to modify eating and lifestyle choices in a way that supports optimum health.

1. **Decline in Basal Metabolic Rate (BMR):**

   - Basal Metabolic Rate, the amount of energy the body needs at rest, tends to decrease with age. This decline is largely attributed to a reduction in lean muscle mass. Since muscle tissue is more metabolically active than fat, a decrease in muscle mass leads to a slower BMR.

2. **Reduction in Muscle Mass:**

   - Sarcopenia, the age-related loss of muscle mass, is a significant contributor to changes in metabolism. As individuals age, there is a decline in the number and size of muscle fibres, impacting the body's ability to burn calories efficiently.

3. **Changes in Body Composition:**

   - Aging is often associated with an increase in body fat and a redistribution of fat from muscle to central areas, such

17

as the abdomen. This shift in body composition further influences metabolic function and can contribute to issues like insulin resistance.

4. **Hormonal Changes:**

   - Hormonal fluctuations play a key role in metabolic changes. For example, there is a decline in growth hormone production, which is essential for maintaining muscle mass. Additionally, changes in thyroid hormone levels and sex hormones can impact metabolism.

5. **Reduced Physical Activity Levels:**

   - With age, there is often a decline in physical activity levels, whether due to changes in mobility, joint issues, or lifestyle factors. Reduced physical activity contributes to the loss of muscle mass and a decrease in overall energy expenditure.

6. **Impaired Nutrient Absorption:**

   - Aging can affect the digestive system, leading to reduced absorption of certain nutrients. Issues such as decreased stomach acid production and changes in gut function may impact the body's ability to extract essential nutrients from food.

7. **Altered Insulin Sensitivity:**

   - Insulin sensitivity tends to decrease with age, leading to a reduced ability of cells to respond to insulin. This can contribute to challenges in blood sugar regulation and an increased risk of conditions like Type 2 diabetes.

8. **Decreased Organ Function:**

- Aging affects the efficiency of various organs, including the liver and kidneys, which play crucial roles in metabolic processes. Changes in organ function can impact the body's ability to metabolize and eliminate substances efficiently.

9. **Hydration Challenges:**

- Aging is associated with a decreased sensation of thirst, leading to potential challenges in maintaining adequate hydration. Dehydration can affect metabolic processes and overall health.

10. **Genetic and Environmental Factors:**

- Genetic predispositions and environmental factors accumulated over a lifetime also contribute to how metabolism changes with age. These factors can influence metabolic rate, body composition, and the overall efficiency of metabolic processes.

Common Metabolic Challenges for Seniors

People experience a variety of physiological changes as they approach senior years, which may have an effect on their metabolic health. These shifts frequently bring with them particular difficulties that need for close observation and customized solutions. Developing solutions to support seniors in maintaining optimal well-being in the face of prevalent metabolic difficulties requires an understanding of these issues.

1. **Sarcopenia and Muscle Loss:**

   - Sarcopenia, the age-related loss of muscle mass, is a prevalent metabolic challenge for seniors. The decline in muscle tissue contributes to a lower basal metabolic rate, making weight management and overall metabolic health more complex.

2. **Reduced Basal Metabolic Rate (BMR):**

   - Seniors often experience a decrease in basal metabolic rate, primarily due to the decline in lean muscle mass. With a lower BMR, the body requires fewer calories at rest, making it easier to gain weight if dietary habits are not adjusted accordingly.

3. **Insulin Resistance and Glucose Regulation:**

   - Aging is associated with changes in insulin sensitivity, leading to an increased risk of insulin resistance. This metabolic challenge can result in difficulties regulating blood sugar levels, potentially contributing to the development of Type 2 diabetes.

4. **Altered Body Composition:**

   - Changes in body composition, characterized by an increase in body fat and a decrease in lean muscle mass, can pose metabolic challenges. This shift may contribute to metabolic syndrome, a cluster of conditions that includes increased blood pressure, high blood sugar, and abnormal cholesterol levels.

5. **Digestive System Changes:**

   - Seniors may experience alterations in the digestive system, such as reduced stomach acid production and changes in gut motility. These changes can impact nutrient absorption, potentially leading to deficiencies and affecting overall metabolic function.

6. **Hydration Issues:**

   - Dehydration becomes a common concern among seniors, partly due to a decreased sense of thirst. Proper hydration is crucial for supporting metabolic processes, and inadequate fluid intake can exacerbate other metabolic challenges.

7. **Hormonal Shifts:**

   - Hormonal changes, including decreases in growth hormone, thyroid hormones, and sex hormones, can influence metabolic function. These shifts may contribute to changes in energy expenditure, body composition, and overall metabolic regulation.

8. **Cardiovascular Health:**

- Aging is associated with an increased risk of cardiovascular issues, such as high blood pressure and elevated cholesterol levels. These factors can impact the cardiovascular system's ability to support efficient metabolic processes.

9. **Bone Health and Calcium Metabolism:**

- Seniors often face challenges related to bone health, including a higher risk of osteoporosis. Changes in calcium metabolism can affect both bone health and overall metabolic equilibrium.

10. **Cognitive Decline:**

- Metabolic challenges can extend to cognitive health, with some studies suggesting a link between metabolic dysfunction and an increased risk of cognitive decline and neurodegenerative disorders in seniors.

11. **Medication Interactions:**

- The use of medications, often common in the senior population, can have metabolic implications. Some medications may impact appetite, nutrient absorption, or directly influence metabolic pathways.

CHAPTER TWO

Lifestyle Habits for Metabolic Health

Incorporating Physical Activity

The foundation of healthy aging is physical activity, which is essential for preserving mobility, averting chronic illnesses, and enhancing general wellbeing. Incorporating physical activity into daily life is crucial for seniors to maintain their independence and to maintain optimal metabolic health.

1. Importance of Physical Activity for Seniors:

- *Maintaining Mobility and Independence:* Regular physical activity helps seniors preserve muscle strength, joint flexibility, and balance, contributing to enhanced mobility and independence in daily activities.

- *Metabolic Health and Weight Management:* Physical activity supports a healthy metabolism by promoting calorie expenditure and preserving lean muscle mass. This is particularly crucial for managing weight and preventing age-related metabolic challenges.

- *Cardiovascular Health:* Aerobic exercises, such as walking or swimming, benefit cardiovascular health by improving circulation, lowering blood pressure, and reducing the risk of heart disease.

- *Bone Health:* Weight-bearing exercises, like walking or resistance training, help maintain bone density and reduce the risk of osteoporosis, a common concern for seniors.

- *Cognitive Function:* Regular physical activity has been linked to better cognitive function and a reduced risk of cognitive decline and neurodegenerative disorders.

- *Mood and Mental Health:* Exercise releases endorphins, promoting a positive mood and reducing the risk of depression and anxiety. Social activities associated with physical activity, such as group classes, also contribute to mental well-being.

2. Types of Physical Activity for Seniors:

- *Aerobic Exercise:* Includes activities like walking, swimming, cycling, and dancing, promoting cardiovascular health and overall endurance.

- *Strength Training:* Involves resistance exercises using weights or resistance bands to build and maintain muscle mass, crucial for functional strength.

- *Flexibility and Balance* Exercises: Activities like yoga or tai chi enhance flexibility and balance, reducing the risk of falls and injuries.

- *Low-Impact Activities:* Gentle exercises like water aerobics or walking are easier on the joints, making them suitable for seniors with mobility issues.

3. Considerations for Seniors:

- *Consultation with Healthcare Professionals:* Before starting a new exercise regimen, seniors should consult with their healthcare provider to ensure that the chosen activities align with their health status and any pre-existing conditions.

- *Gradual Progression:* Seniors should start slowly and gradually increase the intensity and duration of their activities. This approach helps prevent injuries and allows the body to adapt to increased physical demands.

- *Adaptability and Variety:* Physical activity should be adaptable to individual abilities and preferences. Incorporating a variety of exercises keeps routines interesting and targets different aspects of fitness.

- *Hydration and Proper Attire:* Staying hydrated is crucial, especially for seniors. Additionally, wearing appropriate footwear and comfortable clothing helps prevent injuries and enhances the overall exercise experience.

- *Social Engagement:* Joining group activities or classes promotes social engagement, contributing to mental well-being and providing a support system for maintaining regular physical activity.

4. Integration into Daily Life:

- *Routine Walks:* Daily walks, either outdoors or on a treadmill, offer a low-impact yet effective form of aerobic exercise.

- *Home-based Exercises:* Incorporating simple strength and flexibility exercises at home using bodyweight or light resistance can be convenient and effective.

- *Recreational* **Activities:** Participating in recreational activities, such as gardening, dancing, or golfing, provides enjoyable ways to stay active.

- *Technology-Assisted Exercise:* Utilizing fitness apps or following online exercise programs designed for seniors can offer guidance and motivation.

Stress Management and Sleep

Getting enough sleep and managing stress are essential to overall wellbeing, especially for older adults. The ability to manage stress and sustain regular sleep habits becomes more crucial as people age for their physical, mental, and metabolic well-being.

1. Significance of Stress Management for Seniors:

- *Impact on Physical Health:* Chronic stress is associated with various health issues, including cardiovascular problems, immune system suppression, and exacerbation of existing conditions. For seniors, effective stress management is vital to prevent the onset or worsening of age-related health concerns.

- *Cognitive Function:* Stress can negatively affect cognitive function and contribute to memory issues. Managing stress helps in maintaining cognitive sharpness and preventing age-related cognitive decline.

- *Emotional Well-being:* Seniors may face life transitions, health challenges, or loss of loved ones, leading to increased stress. Effective stress management contributes to emotional resilience and a positive outlook on life.

- *Sleep Quality:* Chronic stress can disrupt sleep patterns, making stress management crucial for promoting restful and restorative sleep.

2. Strategies for Stress Management:

- *Mindfulness and Relaxation Techniques*: Practices such as meditation, deep breathing exercises, and progressive muscle relaxation can promote a sense of calm and reduce stress levels.

- *Physical Activity:* Regular physical activity is not only beneficial for metabolic health but also acts as a powerful stress reliever. Activities like walking, yoga, or tai chi can be gentle yet effective.

- *Social Engagement:* Maintaining social connections provides emotional support and opportunities for sharing experiences. Social activities can act as buffers against stress.

- *Hobbies and Leisure Activities:* Engaging in hobbies or leisure activities that bring joy and relaxation helps divert attention from stressors and promotes a sense of fulfilment.

- *Time Management:* Seniors can benefit from effective time management strategies to prioritize tasks and reduce the feeling of being overwhelmed.

- *Counselling or Support Groups:* Seeking professional counselling or participating in support groups can offer a safe space to express feelings and receive guidance on coping with stressors.

3. Significance of Sleep for Seniors:

- *Physical Restoration:* Quality sleep is essential for the body's physical repair processes, including muscle recovery, immune system function, and the release of growth hormone.

- *Cognitive Function and Memory Consolidation:* Adequate sleep supports cognitive functions such as memory consolidation, problem-solving, and decision-making, contributing to overall mental acuity.

- *Mood Regulation:* Sleep plays a crucial role in regulating mood, and seniors who consistently experience good sleep are more likely to maintain emotional well-being.

- *Metabolic Health:* Chronic sleep deprivation is associated with an increased risk of metabolic issues, including insulin resistance and weight gain. Prioritizing sleep is, therefore, crucial for metabolic health in seniors.

4. Strategies for Improving Sleep Quality:

- *Consistent Sleep Schedule:* Maintaining a regular sleep routine by going to bed and waking up at the same time each day helps regulate the body's internal clock.

- ***Creating a Relaxing Bedtime Routine:*** Engaging in calming activities before bedtime, such as reading a book, taking a warm bath, or practicing relaxation techniques, signals to the body that it's time to wind down.

- ***Optimizing Sleep Environment:*** Creating a comfortable and conducive sleep environment involves keeping the bedroom dark, quiet, and cool. Comfortable bedding and a supportive mattress also contribute to sleep quality.

- ***Limiting Stimulants and Electronics:*** Seniors should avoid stimulants like caffeine close to bedtime and limit screen time before sleep, as the blue light emitted from screens can disrupt the natural sleep-wake cycle.

- ***Physical Activity:*** Regular physical activity during the day promotes better sleep. However, strenuous exercise should be avoided close to bedtime.

- ***Healthy Nutrition:*** Maintaining a balanced diet, avoiding heavy meals close to bedtime, and being mindful of food choices can positively impact sleep quality.

CHAPTER THREE

Essential Nutrients for Seniors

Vitamins and Minerals Importance

Vitamins and minerals play crucial roles in maintaining overall health and well-being, and their importance becomes even more pronounced as individuals age. Seniors may face specific nutritional challenges, making a well-balanced intake of vitamins and minerals essential for various bodily functions. Here's a comprehensive discussion on the importance of key vitamins and minerals for seniors:

1. Vitamin D:

- *Bone Health:* Vitamin D is vital for calcium absorption and plays a crucial role in maintaining bone health. Seniors are often at a higher risk of osteoporosis, and sufficient vitamin D levels are essential for preventing fractures and bone-related issues.

- *Immune Function:* Vitamin D also supports immune function, helping seniors better defend against infections and illnesses.

2. Calcium:

- *Bone and Teeth Health:* Calcium is a key mineral for maintaining strong bones and teeth. It becomes particularly important for seniors to prevent the risk of osteoporosis and fractures.

- *Blood Clotting:* Calcium is involved in blood clotting, aiding in wound healing and preventing excessive bleeding.

3. Vitamin B12:

- *Nervous System Health:* Vitamin B12 is crucial for maintaining a healthy nervous system. Seniors may be at a higher risk of B12 deficiency, which can lead to neurological issues, anemia, and fatigue.

- *Energy Production:* B12 is involved in the production of red blood cells and the conversion of food into energy.

4. Vitamin C:

- *Immune Support:* Vitamin C is known for its immune-boosting properties, helping seniors ward off infections and promoting faster recovery.

- *Collagen Production:* Vitamin C is essential for collagen synthesis, contributing to skin health and supporting the integrity of blood vessels, bones, and cartilage.

5. Potassium:

- *Heart Health:* Potassium is crucial for maintaining a healthy balance of fluids in the body and supports proper heart function. It helps regulate blood pressure and reduces the risk of cardiovascular issues.

- *Muscle Function:* Adequate potassium levels are necessary for proper muscle contraction, making it important for mobility and preventing muscle cramps.

6. Magnesium:

- *Bone Health:* Magnesium works in conjunction with calcium for bone health and may help reduce the risk of osteoporosis.

- *Heart Health:* Magnesium is involved in maintaining a regular heartbeat and supporting overall cardiovascular health.

- *Muscle Function:* Adequate magnesium levels contribute to proper muscle function and may help alleviate muscle cramps.

7. Vitamin K:

- *Blood Clotting:* Vitamin K is essential for blood clotting and wound healing. It also plays a role in bone metabolism.

- *Bone Health:* Vitamin K is involved in the regulation of calcium, contributing to bone density and reducing the risk of fractures.

8. Folate (Vitamin B9):

- *Brain Health:* Folate is important for brain health and cognitive function. It plays a role in neurotransmitter synthesis and may contribute to the prevention of age-related cognitive decline.

- *Cell Division:* Folate is crucial for DNA synthesis and cell division, making it essential for overall growth and development.

9. Iron:

- *Oxygen Transport:* Iron is a component of hemoglobin, the protein in red blood cells that carries oxygen to tissues. Sufficient iron levels prevent anemia and support energy levels.

- *Immune Function:* Iron is involved in immune function, aiding in the body's defence against infections.

10. Zinc:

- *Immune Support:* Zinc is vital for immune function, supporting the body's ability to fight off infections and illnesses.

- *Wound Healing:* Zinc plays a role in wound healing and helps maintain the integrity of the skin.

11. Omega-3 Fatty Acids:

- *Heart Health:* Omega-3 fatty acids, including EPA and DHA, support cardiovascular health by reducing inflammation, improving cholesterol levels, and maintaining blood vessel health.

- *Brain Health:* Omega-3s are essential for brain health and may contribute to cognitive function, potentially reducing the risk of age-related cognitive decline.

Hydration Tips for Metabolic Health

Proper hydration is a foundational element of overall health and becomes increasingly critical as individuals age. Hydration plays a pivotal role in supporting metabolic health, cognitive function, and various physiological processes. For seniors, maintaining optimal hydration levels is essential to promote well-being. Here are professional hydration tips specifically tailored for metabolic health in seniors:

1. Awareness of Individual Hydration Needs:

- Recognize that hydration needs vary based on factors such as age, weight, activity level, and health status. Seniors should be encouraged to stay attuned to their individual hydration requirements.

2. Regular Water Intake:

- Emphasize the importance of regular water consumption throughout the day. Encourage seniors to sip water consistently rather than relying on infrequent large quantities. Adequate hydration supports metabolic processes and helps prevent dehydration-related issues.

3. Monitor Urine Colour:

- Urine colour is an effective indicator of hydration status. Encourage seniors to monitor the colour of their urine; a pale yellow colour suggests proper hydration, while darker shades may indicate dehydration.

4. Hydrating Foods:

- Incorporate hydrating foods into the diet. Fruits and vegetables with high water content, such as watermelon, cucumber, and oranges, not only contribute to fluid intake but also provide essential vitamins and minerals.

5. Set Hydration Goals:

- Establish daily hydration goals tailored to individual needs. Seniors can use a water bottle with marked measurements to track their daily water intake, making it easier to achieve and maintain optimal hydration levels.

6. Include Electrolytes:

- In certain situations, especially during physical activity or hot weather, consider the inclusion of beverages containing electrolytes. This helps restore electrolyte balance and supports metabolic processes.

7. Be Mindful of Medications:

- Some medications may contribute to increased fluid loss or affect thirst perception. Seniors should be aware of the potential impact of medications on hydration and consult with healthcare professionals if adjustments are needed.

8. Hydration and Exercise:

- Encourage seniors to hydrate before, during, and after physical activity. Proper hydration supports energy levels, helps regulate body temperature, and enhances the overall effectiveness of exercise.

9. Monitor Fluid Intake in Extreme Temperatures:

- In hot or cold climates, seniors are more susceptible to dehydration. Increased fluid intake is crucial during extreme temperatures to prevent dehydration-related complications and support metabolic resilience.

10. Hydration and Cognitive Function:

- Emphasize the connection between hydration and cognitive function. Proper fluid intake helps maintain mental clarity, focus, and overall cognitive well-being, which is especially important for seniors.

11. Limit Caffeine and Alcohol:

- Both caffeine and alcohol can contribute to dehydration. Seniors should be mindful of their intake of caffeinated and alcoholic beverages and balance them with an increased intake of water.

12. Address Hydration Challenges:

- Recognize potential challenges to hydration, such as reduced thirst perception, and proactively address them. Establishing a routine for regular water consumption, even in the absence of thirst cues, is essential for maintaining hydration.

BREAKFAST RECIPES

Quinoa Breakfast Bowl

A protein-packed and fiber-rich breakfast to kickstart the day, promoting sustained energy levels and supporting metabolic function.

Ingredients: 1/2 cup quinoa, rinsed

- 1 cup almond milk
- 1/2 cup mixed berries
- 1 tablespoon chia seeds
- 1 tablespoon sliced almonds
- 1 teaspoon honey

Prep Time: 5 minutes

Cooking Time: 15 minutes

Serving Size: 1

Serving Time: Morning

Nutritional Information (per serving):

- Calories: 350
- Protein: 12g
- Fiber: 8g
- Healthy Fats: 10g

Directions:

1. In a saucepan, combine quinoa and almond milk. Bring to a boil, then reduce heat and simmer for 15 minutes until quinoa is cooked.
2. Transfer cooked quinoa to a bowl and top with mixed berries, chia seeds, sliced almonds, and a drizzle of honey.

Serving Methods:

- Serve warm with a dollop of Greek yogurt.

- Sprinkle with a pinch of cinnamon for added flavor.

Greek Yogurt Parfait

A delicious and protein-rich breakfast, perfect for supporting muscle health and providing essential nutrients.

Ingredients:

- 1 cup Greek yogurt
- 1/2 cup granola (low sugar)
- 1/2 cup fresh fruit (e.g., sliced strawberries, blueberries)
- 1 tablespoon chopped nuts (e.g., walnuts, almonds)
- 1 teaspoon honey

Prep Time: 5 minutes

Serving Size: 1

Serving Time: Morning

Nutritional Information (per serving):

- Calories: 400
- Protein: 20g
- Fiber: 6g
- Healthy Fats: 10g

Directions:

1. In a glass or bowl, layer Greek yogurt, granola, fresh fruit, and chopped nuts.
2. Drizzle with honey for added sweetness.

Serving Methods:

- Experiment with different fruit combinations based on seasonal availability.
- Add a sprinkle of flaxseeds for an extra boost of omega-3 fatty acids.

Spinach and Feta Omelette

Packed with protein and nutrients, this omelette provides a savory and satisfying option for a metabolic-boosting breakfast.

Ingredients:

- 2 large eggs
- 1/2 cup fresh spinach, chopped
- 2 tablespoons feta cheese, crumbled
- 1 tablespoon olive oil
- Salt and pepper to taste
- Fresh herbs for garnish (e.g., parsley)

Prep Time: 7 minutes

Cooking Time: 5 minutes

Serving Size: 1

Serving Time: Morning

Nutritional Information (per serving):

- Calories: 320
- Protein: 18g
- Fiber: 2g
- Healthy Fats: 25g

Directions:

1. In a bowl, whisk eggs and season with salt and pepper.
2. Heat olive oil in a non-stick pan, add chopped spinach, and sauté until wilted.
3. Pour whisked eggs over the spinach, add crumbled feta, and cook until set.
4. Fold the omelette, garnish with fresh herbs, and serve.

Serving Methods:

- Pair with a side of whole-grain toast.

- Serve with a slice of avocado for added creaminess.

Chia Seed Pudding with Berries

A nutrient-dense and fiber-rich pudding providing a satisfying and delicious start to the day.

Ingredients:

- 2 tablespoons chia seeds
- 1 cup almond milk
- 1/2 teaspoon vanilla extract
- 1 tablespoon maple syrup
- 1/2 cup mixed berries

Prep Time: 5 minutes (plus chilling time)

Serving Size: 1

Serving Time: Morning

Nutritional Information (per serving):

- Calories: 250
- Protein: 7g
- Fiber: 10g
- Healthy Fats: 8g

Directions:

1. In a bowl, mix chia seeds, almond milk, vanilla extract, and maple syrup. Stir well and refrigerate for at least 2 hours or overnight.
2. Top with mixed berries before serving.

Serving Methods:

- Add a sprinkle of crushed nuts for added crunch.
- Garnish with a mint leaf for freshness.

Whole-Grain Pancakes with Banana and Walnuts

A wholesome and heart-healthy pancake recipe incorporating whole grains, fruits, and nuts for a nutritious and filling breakfast.

Ingredients:

- 1/2 cup whole-grain pancake mix
- 1/3 cup water or almond milk
- 1/2 ripe banana, mashed
- 1 tablespoon chopped walnuts
- 1 teaspoon honey

Prep Time: 10 minutes

Cooking Time: 8 minutes

Serving Size: 2 pancakes

Serving Time: Morning

Nutritional Information (per serving):

- Calories: 280
- Protein: 8g
- Fiber: 5g
- Healthy Fats: 7g

Directions:

1. In a bowl, mix pancake mix and water or almond milk until smooth.
2. Fold in mashed banana and chopped walnuts.
3. Heat a non-stick pan and ladle the batter to make pancakes. Cook until bubbles appear, flip, and cook the other side.
4. Drizzle with honey before serving.

Serving Methods:

- Top with a dollop of Greek yogurt.
- Serve with a side of fresh berries for added antioxidants.

Avocado and Salmon Toast

A nutrient-dense and omega-3 rich toast that combines the creaminess of avocado with the health benefits of salmon.

Ingredients:

- 1 slice whole-grain bread
- 1/2 ripe avocado, mashed
- 2 ounces smoked salmon
- 1 teaspoon capers
- Lemon wedge for garnish

Prep Time: 5 minutes

Serving Size: 1

Serving Time: Morning

Nutritional Information (per serving):

- Calories: 320
- Protein: 15g
- Fiber: 6g
- Healthy Fats: 18g

Directions:

1. Toast the whole-grain bread until golden brown.
2. Spread mashed avocado on the toast and layer with smoked salmon.
3. Sprinkle capers on top and garnish with a squeeze of lemon.

Serving Methods:

- Add a sprinkle of black pepper for extra flavor.
- Serve with a side of mixed greens for added freshness.

Blueberry and Almond Smoothie Bowl

A refreshing and antioxidant-rich smoothie bowl combining blueberries, almonds, and Greek yogurt for a satisfying and nutritious breakfast.

Ingredients:

- 1 cup frozen blueberries
- 1/2 cup almond milk
- 1/2 banana
- 1/4 cup Greek yogurt
- 1 tablespoon almond butter
- Toppings: sliced almonds, chia seeds, fresh blueberries

Prep Time: 5 minutes

Serving Size: 1

Serving Time: Morning

Nutritional Information (per serving):

- Calories: 350
- Protein: 12g
- Fiber: 8g
- Healthy Fats: 15g

Directions:

1. Blend frozen blueberries, almond milk, banana, Greek yogurt, and almond butter until smooth.
2. Pour into a bowl and top with sliced almonds, chia seeds, and fresh blueberries.

Serving Methods:

- Customize with additional toppings such as shredded coconut or granola.
- Drizzle with honey for added sweetness.

Sweet Potato and Kale Breakfast Hash

A nutrient-dense and fiber-rich breakfast hash that combines the goodness of sweet potatoes, kale, and eggs for a satisfying morning meal.

Ingredients: 1 small sweet potato, diced

- 1 cup kale, chopped
- 2 eggs
- 1 tablespoon olive oil
- Salt and pepper to taste

Prep Time: 10 minutes

Cooking Time: 15 minutes

Serving Size: 1

Serving Time: Morning

Nutritional Information (per serving):

- Calories: 300
- Protein: 14g
- Fiber: 6g
- Healthy Fats: 12g

Directions:

1. In a skillet, heat olive oil and sauté diced sweet potatoes until they begin to soften.
2. Add chopped kale and continue cooking until sweet potatoes are cooked through and kale is wilted.
3. Make two wells in the hash and crack eggs into them. Cover and cook until eggs are done to your liking.

Serving Methods:

- Top with a sprinkle of feta cheese.
- Serve with a side of sliced avocado for added creaminess.

Oatmeal with Apples and Cinnamon

A heart-healthy and fiber-rich oatmeal topped with apples and cinnamon for a comforting and nutritious breakfast.

Ingredients:

- 1/2 cup old-fashioned oats
- 1 cup water or almond milk
- 1 small apple, diced
- 1/2 teaspoon cinnamon
- 1 tablespoon chopped walnuts
- 1 teaspoon maple syrup

Prep Time: 5 minutes

Cooking Time: 5 minutes

Serving Size: 1

Serving Time: Morning

Nutritional Information (per serving):

- Calories: 280
- Protein: 7g
- Fiber: 8g
- Healthy Fats: 10g

Directions:

1. In a saucepan, combine oats and water or almond milk. Cook until oats are soft and the mixture thickens.
2. Stir in diced apples, cinnamon, and chopped walnuts.
3. Drizzle with maple syrup before serving.

Serving Methods:

- Add a dollop of Greek yogurt for extra creaminess.
- Sprinkle with ground flaxseeds for additional fiber.

Egg and Vegetable Breakfast Wrap

A protein-packed and fiber-rich breakfast wrap with eggs and colorful vegetables for a nutritious and portable morning meal.

Ingredients:

- 2 whole eggs, beaten
- 1 whole-grain wrap
- 1/2 cup mixed vegetables (bell peppers, spinach, tomatoes)
- 1 tablespoon feta cheese, crumbled
- Salt and pepper to taste
- Fresh herbs for garnish (e.g., cilantro)

Prep Time: 10 minutes

Cooking Time: 5 minutes

Serving Size: 1

Serving Time: Morning

Nutritional Information (per serving):

- Calories: 320
- Protein: 18g
- Fiber: 6g
- Healthy Fats: 12g

Directions:

1. In a pan, sauté mixed vegetables until tender.
2. Pour beaten eggs over the vegetables, scramble until cooked.
3. Place the egg and vegetable mixture on a whole-grain wrap, **sprinkle with crumbled feta, and garnish with fresh herbs.**

Serving Methods:

- Serve with a side of salsa for added flavor.
- Wrap in parchment paper for an on-the-go breakfast option.

Blueberry Almond Overnight Oats

A convenient and nutritious breakfast that combines the goodness of oats, blueberries, and almonds. Overnight oats are soaked overnight for a no-fuss morning meal.

Ingredients:

- 1/2 cup old-fashioned oats
- 1/2 cup almond milk
- 1/2 cup fresh blueberries
- 1 tablespoon almond slices
- 1 teaspoon honey

Prep Time: 5 minutes

Serving Size: 1

Serving Time: Morning

Nutritional Information (per serving):

- Calories: 300
- Protein: 8g
- Fiber: 6g
- Healthy Fats: 10g

Directions:

1. In a jar, combine oats, almond milk, and blueberries.
2. Refrigerate overnight.
3. In the morning, top with almond slices and drizzle with honey.

Serving Methods:

- Add a dollop of Greek yogurt.
- Sprinkle with a pinch of cinnamon for extra flavor.

Veggie Egg Muffins

Protein-packed egg muffins with colorful veggies make for a delicious and customizable breakfast, supporting metabolic health.

Ingredients:

- 2 eggs, beaten
- 1/4 cup bell peppers, diced
- 1/4 cup spinach, chopped
- 1/4 cup cherry tomatoes, halved
- 1 tablespoon feta cheese, crumbled

Prep Time: 10 minutes

Cooking Time: 15 minutes

Serving Size: 2 muffins

Serving Time: Morning

Nutritional Information (per serving):

- Calories: 220
- Protein: 14g
- Fiber: 2g
- Healthy Fats: 12g

Directions:

1. Preheat the oven to 350°F (175°C).
2. In a bowl, mix beaten eggs, bell peppers, spinach, and cherry tomatoes.
3. Pour the mixture into muffin cups, top with crumbled feta, and bake for 15 minutes.

Serving Methods:

- Serve with a side of whole-grain toast.
- Top with a dollop of salsa for added flavor.

Cinnamon Apple Quinoa Porridge

A warm and comforting quinoa porridge with cinnamon and apples, providing a nutritious and satisfying start to the day.

Ingredients:

- 1/2 cup quinoa, rinsed
- 1 cup water or almond milk
- 1/2 apple, diced
- 1/2 teaspoon cinnamon
- 1 tablespoon chopped walnuts
- 1 teaspoon maple syrup

Prep Time: 10 minutes

Cooking Time: 15 minutes

Serving Size: 1

Serving Time: Morning

Nutritional Information (per serving):

- Calories: 320
- Protein: 10g
- Fiber: 6g
- Healthy Fats: 8g

Directions:

1. In a saucepan, combine quinoa and water or almond milk. Bring to a boil, then simmer for 15 minutes.
2. Stir in diced apples, cinnamon, and chopped walnuts.
3. Drizzle with maple syrup before serving.

Serving Methods:

- Top with a spoonful of Greek yogurt.
- Garnish with a sprinkle of ground flaxseeds.

Smoked Salmon and Avocado Bagel

A sophisticated yet simple breakfast featuring the classic combination of smoked salmon and creamy avocado on a whole-grain bagel.

Ingredients: 1 whole-grain bagel, toasted

- 2 ounces smoked salmon
- 1/2 avocado, sliced
- 1 tablespoon cream cheese
- Lemon wedge for garnish

Prep Time: 5 minutes

Serving Size: 1

Serving Time: Morning

Nutritional Information (per serving):

- Calories: 350, Protein: 20g
- Fiber: 6g
- Healthy Fats: 15g

Directions:

1. Toast the whole-grain bagel until golden brown.
2. Spread cream cheese on the bagel halves and layer with smoked salmon and avocado slices.
3. Garnish with a squeeze of lemon.

Serving Methods:

- Add a sprinkle of capers for extra flavor.
- Serve with a side of mixed greens for freshness.

Quinoa and Berry Breakfast Parfait

A visually appealing and nutrient-packed parfait combining layers of quinoa, Greek yogurt, and fresh berries for a delightful morning treat.

Ingredients: 1/2 cup cooked quinoa

- 1/2 cup Greek yogurt

- 1/2 cup mixed berries (strawberries, blueberries)
- 1 tablespoon honey
- 1 tablespoon sliced almonds

Prep Time: 10 minutes

Serving Size: 1

Serving Time: Morning

Nutritional Information (per serving):

- Calories: 280
- Protein: 15g
- Fiber: 5g
- Healthy Fats: 8g

Directions:

1. In a glass or bowl, layer cooked quinoa, Greek yogurt, and mixed berries.
2. Drizzle with honey and sprinkle with sliced almonds.

Serving Methods:

- Add a pinch of cinnamon for additional warmth.
- Include a spoonful of chia seeds for extra fiber.

Banana Walnut Breakfast Smoothie

A nutrient-rich and filling smoothie featuring the natural sweetness of bananas and the crunch of walnuts for a balanced breakfast option.

Ingredients: 1 banana

- 1/2 cup plain Greek yogurt
- 1/4 cup rolled oats
- 1 tablespoon chopped walnuts
- 1/2 cup almond milk
- Ice cubes (optional)

Prep Time: 5 minutes

Serving Size: 1

Serving Time: Morning

Nutritional Information (per serving):

- Calories: 320
- Protein: 15g
- Fiber: 5g
- Healthy Fats: 10g

Directions:

1. In a blender, combine banana, Greek yogurt, rolled oats, chopped walnuts, and almond milk.
2. Blend until smooth. Add ice cubes if desired.

Serving Methods:

- Garnish with a sprinkle of cinnamon for added flavor.
- Top with a few whole walnuts for a crunchy texture.

Sweet Potato and Kale Frittata

A savory and nutrient-packed frittata featuring sweet potatoes and kale, providing a wholesome and satisfying breakfast.

Ingredients:

- 2 eggs, beaten
- 1/2 cup sweet potatoes, diced
- 1 cup kale, chopped
- 1 tablespoon feta cheese, crumbled
- 1 tablespoon olive oil
- Salt and pepper to taste

Prep Time: 10 minutes

Cooking Time: 15 minutes

Serving Size: 1

Serving Time: Morning

Nutritional Information (per serving):

- Calories: 300
- Protein: 14g
- Fiber: 4g
- Healthy Fats: 15g

Directions:

1. Preheat the oven to 350°F (175°C).
2. In an oven-safe skillet, sauté sweet potatoes in olive oil until slightly tender.
3. Add chopped kale and cook until wilted.
4. Pour beaten eggs over the vegetables, top with crumbled feta, and bake for 15 minutes.

Serving Methods:

- Serve with a side of sliced avocado.
- Garnish with fresh herbs such as parsley.

Berry Protein Pancakes

A protein-packed pancake recipe featuring the goodness of berries, providing a delicious and energizing breakfast.

Ingredients:

- 1/2 cup whole-grain pancake mix
- 1/3 cup water or almond milk
- 1/2 cup mixed berries (strawberries, blueberries)
- 1 tablespoon Greek yogurt
- 1 teaspoon maple syrup

Prep Time: 10 minutes

Cooking Time: 8 minutes

Serving Size: 2 pancakes

Serving Time: Morning

Nutritional Information (per serving):

- Calories: 280
- Protein: 10g
- Fiber: 4g
- Healthy Fats: 5g

Directions:

1. In a bowl, mix pancake mix and water or almond milk until smooth.
2. Fold in mixed berries.
3. Heat a non-stick pan and ladle the batter to make pancakes. Cook until bubbles appear, flip, and cook the other side.
4. Top with Greek yogurt and drizzle with maple syrup.

Serving Methods:

- Sprinkle with a handful of granola for added crunch.
- Serve with a side of fresh fruit for extra sweetness.

Mediterranean Egg Wrap

A flavorful and Mediterranean-inspired egg wrap with tomatoes, olives, and feta, offering a unique and nutritious breakfast experience.

Ingredients:

- 2 whole eggs, beaten
- 1 whole-grain wrap
- 1/4 cup cherry tomatoes, halved
- 2 tablespoons black olives, sliced
- 1 tablespoon feta cheese, crumbled
- Fresh basil for garnish

Prep Time: 10 minutes

Cooking Time: 5 minutes

Serving Size: 1

Serving Time: Morning

Nutritional Information (per serving):

- Calories: 320
- Protein: 16g
- Fiber: 5g
- Healthy Fats: 12g

Directions:

1. In a pan, scramble beaten eggs until cooked.
2. Warm the whole-grain wrap.
3. Fill the wrap with scrambled eggs, cherry tomatoes, sliced olives, and crumbled feta.
4. Garnish with fresh basil.

Serving Methods:

- Drizzle with extra virgin olive oil for added richness.
- Serve with a side of mixed greens.

Pumpkin Spice Chia Seed Pudding

A seasonal and nutrient-rich chia seed pudding infused with pumpkin spice, offering a delightful and healthy breakfast option.

Ingredients:

- 2 tablespoons chia seeds
- 1 cup unsweetened almond milk
- 1/4 cup pumpkin puree
- 1/2 teaspoon pumpkin spice
- 1 tablespoon chopped pecans
- 1 teaspoon maple syrup

Prep Time: 5 minutes (plus chilling time)

Serving Size: 1

Serving Time: Morning

Nutritional Information (per serving):

- Calories: 250

- Protein: 7g
- Fiber: 10g
- Healthy Fats: 8g

Directions:

1. In a bowl, mix chia seeds, almond milk, pumpkin puree, and pumpkin spice. Stir well and refrigerate for at least 2 hours or overnight.
2. Top with chopped pecans and drizzle with maple syrup before serving.

Serving Methods:

- Garnish with a dollop of coconut whipped cream.
- Sprinkle with a pinch of cinnamon for extra warmth.

Grilled Chicken Salad with Citrus Vinaigrette

A light and refreshing salad with grilled chicken, mixed greens, and a zesty citrus vinaigrette, providing a balanced and flavorful lunch option.

Ingredients: 4 oz grilled chicken breast, sliced

- 2 cups mixed salad greens, 1/2 cup cherry tomatoes, halved
- 1/4 cup cucumber, sliced
- 1/4 cup red bell pepper, diced
- Citrus Vinaigrette: 2 tablespoons olive oil, 1 tablespoon orange juice, 1 tablespoon lemon juice, salt, and pepper to taste

Prep Time: 15 minutes

Cooking Time: 10 minutes (for grilling chicken)

Serving Size: 1

Serving Time: Lunch

Nutritional Information (per serving):

- Calories: 350
- Protein: 25g
- Fiber: 5g
- Healthy Fats: 20g

Directions:

1. Grill chicken breast until fully cooked, then slice.
2. In a large bowl, combine salad greens, cherry tomatoes, cucumber, and red bell pepper.
3. Top with grilled chicken slices.
4. Whisk together the ingredients for the citrus vinaigrette and drizzle over the salad.

Serving Methods:

- Serve with a side of whole-grain bread.

- Add a sprinkle of feta cheese for extra flavor.

Salmon and Quinoa Stuffed Bell Peppers

A protein-packed and nutrient-dense dish where bell peppers are stuffed with a delicious mixture of salmon, quinoa, and vegetables, creating a satisfying lunch.

Ingredients:

- 2 bell peppers, halved and seeds removed
- 6 oz salmon fillet, cooked and flaked
- 1/2 cup cooked quinoa
- 1/4 cup black beans, drained and rinsed
- 1/4 cup corn kernels
- 1/4 cup cherry tomatoes, diced
- 1 tablespoon fresh cilantro, chopped
- 1/2 teaspoon cumin
- Salt and pepper to taste

Prep Time: 20 minutes

Cooking Time: 20 minutes (includes baking time)

Serving Size: 2 halves

Serving Time: Lunch

Nutritional Information (per serving):

- Calories: 400
- Protein: 25g
- Fiber: 8g
- Healthy Fats: 15g

Directions:

1. Preheat the oven to 375°F (190°C).
2. In a bowl, mix together flaked salmon, cooked quinoa, black beans, corn, cherry tomatoes, cilantro, cumin, salt, and pepper.
3. Stuff the bell pepper halves with the salmon and quinoa mixture.

4. Bake for 20 minutes or until peppers are tender.

Serving Methods:

- Drizzle with a yogurt-based sauce.
- Serve with a side of mixed greens.

Mushroom and Spinach Quiche

A savory quiche filled with mushrooms, spinach, and a light egg custard, offering a delicious and protein-rich lunch option.

Ingredients:

- 1 pre-made whole-grain pie crust
- 1 cup mushrooms, sliced
- 1 cup fresh spinach, chopped
- 4 large eggs
- 1 cup milk (dairy or plant-based)
- 1/2 cup Swiss cheese, grated
- Salt and pepper to taste
- Pinch of nutmeg

Prep Time: 15 minutes

Cooking Time: 40 minutes (includes baking time)

Serving Size: 1 slice

Serving Time: Lunch

Nutritional Information (per serving):

- Calories: 280
- Protein: 14g
- Fiber: 3g
- Healthy Fats: 15g

Directions:

1. Preheat the oven to 375°F (190°C).
2. In a skillet, sauté mushrooms and spinach until softened.

3. In a bowl, whisk together eggs, milk, Swiss cheese, salt, pepper, and nutmeg.
4. Place the pre-made pie crust in a pie dish, add the sautéed vegetables, and pour the egg mixture over.
5. Bake for 40 minutes or until the quiche is set.

Serving Methods:

- Serve with a side of mixed greens.
- Enjoy with a dollop of Greek yogurt.

Turkey and Vegetable Stir-Fry with Brown Rice

A quick and nutritious stir-fry featuring lean turkey, colorful vegetables, and brown rice, providing a well-balanced and flavorful lunch.

Ingredients:

- 8 oz lean ground turkey
- 1 cup broccoli florets
- 1/2 cup bell peppers, sliced
- 1/2 cup carrots, julienned
- 2 tablespoons low-sodium soy sauce
- 1 tablespoon hoisin sauce
- 1 teaspoon sesame oil
- 1 cup cooked brown rice

Prep Time: 15 minutes

Cooking Time: 15 minutes

Serving Size: 1

Serving Time: Lunch

Nutritional Information (per serving):

- Calories: 380
- Protein: 25g
- Fiber: 6g
- Healthy Fats: 10g

Directions:

1. In a wok or skillet, brown ground turkey until fully cooked.
2. Add broccoli, bell peppers, and carrots to the skillet and stir-fry until vegetables are tender-crisp.
3. In a small bowl, mix soy sauce, hoisin sauce, and sesame oil. Pour over the turkey and vegetable mixture.
4. Serve over cooked brown rice.

Serving Methods:

- Garnish with sliced green onions.
- Add a sprinkle of sesame seeds for extra crunch.

Caprese Chicken Wrap

A light and satisfying wrap featuring grilled chicken, fresh tomatoes, mozzarella, and basil, creating a classic Caprese flavor combination.

Ingredients:

- 4 oz grilled chicken breast, sliced
- 1 whole-grain wrap
- 1/2 cup cherry tomatoes, halved
- 1/4 cup fresh mozzarella, sliced
- Fresh basil leaves
- Balsamic glaze for drizzling

Prep Time: 15 minutes

Cooking Time: 10 minutes (for grilling chicken)

Serving Size: 1

Serving Time: Lunch

Nutritional Information (per serving):

- Calories: 340
- Protein: 30g
- Fiber: 5g
- Healthy Fats: 15g

Directions:

1. Grill chicken breast until fully cooked, then slice.
2. Warm the whole-grain wrap.
3. Layer sliced chicken, cherry tomatoes, fresh mozzarella, and basil leaves on the wrap.
4. Drizzle with balsamic glaze before rolling up.

Serving Methods:

- Serve with a side of mixed greens.
- Add a spread of pesto for extra flavor.

Lentil and Vegetable Soup

A hearty and fiber-rich soup featuring lentils, assorted vegetables, and flavorful herbs, providing a nourishing and comforting lunch.

Ingredients:

- 1 cup dry lentils, rinsed and drained
- 4 cups vegetable broth
- 1 cup carrots, diced
- 1 cup celery, diced
- 1 cup onion, diced
- 2 cloves garlic, minced
- 1 teaspoon dried thyme
- 1 teaspoon dried rosemary
- Salt and pepper to taste

Prep Time: 15 minutes

Cooking Time: 30 minutes

Serving Size: 2 cups

Serving Time: Lunch

Nutritional Information (per serving):

- Calories: 280
- Protein: 18g

- Fiber: 10g
- Healthy Fats: 2g

Directions:

1. In a large pot, combine lentils, vegetable broth, carrots, celery, onion, garlic, thyme, and rosemary.
2. Bring to a boil, then simmer for 30 minutes or until lentils are tender.
3. Season with salt and pepper to taste.

Serving Methods:

- Sprinkle with chopped fresh parsley.
- Serve with a slice of whole-grain bread.

Shrimp and Quinoa Bowl

A protein-rich and flavorful bowl featuring succulent shrimp, quinoa, and a medley of vegetables, offering a satisfying and well-balanced lunch.

Ingredients:

- 8 oz shrimp, peeled and deveined
- 1/2 cup cooked quinoa
- 1 cup broccoli florets
- 1/2 cup snap peas, halved
- 1/4 cup red bell pepper, sliced
- 1 tablespoon olive oil
- 1 tablespoon soy sauce
- 1 teaspoon sesame seeds

Prep Time: 20 minutes

Cooking Time: 10 minutes

Serving Size: 1

Serving Time: Lunch

Nutritional Information (per serving):

- Calories: 320

- Protein: 22g
- Fiber: 5g
- Healthy Fats: 12g

Directions:

1. In a skillet, heat olive oil and sauté shrimp until pink and opaque.
2. Add broccoli, snap peas, and red bell pepper. Stir-fry until vegetables are tender-crisp.
3. Stir in cooked quinoa and soy sauce. Cook for an additional 2 minutes.
4. Sprinkle with sesame seeds before serving.

Serving Methods:

- Garnish with chopped green onions.
- Drizzle with a squeeze of lime for freshness.

Mediterranean Chickpea Salad

A vibrant and protein-packed salad featuring chickpeas, tomatoes, cucumbers, and feta, tossed in a Mediterranean-inspired dressing for a refreshing lunch.

Ingredients:

- 1 can (15 oz) chickpeas, drained and rinsed
- 1 cup cherry tomatoes, halved
- 1/2 cucumber, diced
- 1/4 cup red onion, finely chopped
- 2 tablespoons feta cheese, crumbled
- Dressing: 2 tablespoons olive oil, 1 tablespoon red wine vinegar, 1 teaspoon dried oregano, salt, and pepper to taste

Prep Time: 15 minutes

Serving Size: 2

Serving Time: Lunch

Nutritional Information (per serving):

- Calories: 280
- Protein: 12g
- Fiber: 8g
- Healthy Fats: 14g

Directions:

1. In a bowl, combine chickpeas, cherry tomatoes, cucumber, red onion, and feta cheese.
2. In a separate bowl, whisk together olive oil, red wine vinegar, dried oregano, salt, and pepper.
3. Pour the dressing over the salad and toss to combine.

Serving Methods:

- Serve over a bed of mixed greens.
- Enjoy with a side of whole-grain pita.

Turkey and Veggie Wrap with Hummus

A satisfying wrap featuring lean turkey, assorted vegetables, and creamy hummus, providing a nutrient-rich and flavorful lunch.

Ingredients:

- 4 oz lean turkey slices
- 1 whole-grain wrap
- 1/2 cup spinach leaves
- 1/4 cup cherry tomatoes, halved
- 1/4 cup cucumber, sliced
- 2 tablespoons hummus

Prep Time: 10 minutes

Serving Size: 1

Serving Time: Lunch

Nutritional Information (per serving):

- Calories: 320
- Protein: 20g

- Fiber: 5g
- Healthy Fats: 12g

Directions:

1. Lay the whole-grain wrap flat.
2. Layer turkey slices, spinach leaves, cherry tomatoes, cucumber, and hummus on the wrap.
3. Roll up tightly.

Serving Methods:

- Cut into bite-sized pinwheels for easy serving.
- Add a sprinkle of black pepper for extra flavor.

Vegetarian Stuffed Bell Peppers

A wholesome and colorful dish where bell peppers are stuffed with a mix of quinoa, black beans, corn, and spices, offering a satisfying and meatless lunch.

Ingredients:

- 2 bell peppers, halved and seeds removed
- 1/2 cup cooked quinoa
- 1/2 cup black beans, drained and rinsed
- 1/4 cup corn kernels
- 1/4 cup red onion, finely chopped
- 1 teaspoon cumin
- 1/2 teaspoon chili powder
- Salt and pepper to taste

Prep Time: 20 minutes

Cooking Time: 25 minutes (includes baking time)

Serving Size: 2 halves

Serving Time: Lunch

Nutritional Information (per serving):

- Calories: 300

- Protein: 12g
- Fiber: 8g
- Healthy Fats: 5g

Directions:

1. Preheat the oven to 375°F (190°C).
2. In a bowl, mix together cooked quinoa, black beans, corn, red onion, cumin, chili powder, salt, and pepper.
3. Stuff the bell pepper halves with the quinoa and black bean mixture.
4. Bake for 25 minutes or until peppers are tender.

Serving Methods:

- Top with a dollop of Greek yogurt.
- Serve with a side of salsa for added flavor.

Quinoa and Vegetable Stir-Fry

A vibrant and nutritious stir-fry that combines protein-rich quinoa with a colorful assortment of vegetables, providing a satisfying and well-balanced lunch.

Ingredients:

- 1 cup cooked quinoa
- 1/2 cup broccoli florets
- 1/2 cup bell peppers, sliced
- 1/2 cup snap peas, halved
- 1/4 cup carrots, julienned
- 2 tablespoons low-sodium soy sauce
- 1 tablespoon sesame oil
- 1 teaspoon ginger, minced
- 1 clove garlic, minced

Prep Time: 15 minutes

Cooking Time: 10 minutes

Serving Size: 1

Serving Time: Lunch

Nutritional Information (per serving):

- Calories: 320
- Protein: 12g
- Fiber: 8g
- Healthy Fats: 10g

Directions:

1. In a wok or skillet, heat sesame oil and sauté garlic and ginger until fragrant.
2. Add broccoli, bell peppers, snap peas, and carrots. Stir-fry until vegetables are tender-crisp.
3. Stir in cooked quinoa and soy sauce. Cook for an additional 2 minutes.
4. Serve hot.

Serving Methods:

- Garnish with sesame seeds for added crunch.
- Top with a drizzle of teriyaki sauce for extra flavor.

Turkey and Lentil Soup

A hearty and protein-packed soup featuring lean turkey, lentils, and a medley of vegetables, offering a comforting and nutritious lunch.

Ingredients:

- 8 oz lean ground turkey
- 1 cup dry lentils, rinsed and drained
- 4 cups low-sodium chicken broth
- 1 cup carrots, diced
- 1/2 cup celery, diced
- 1/2 cup onion, diced
- 2 cloves garlic, minced
- 1 teaspoon dried thyme
- Salt and pepper to taste

Prep Time: 20 minutes

Cooking Time: 30 minutes

Serving Size: 2 cups

Serving Time: Lunch

Nutritional Information (per serving):

- Calories: 350
- Protein: 25g
- Fiber: 12g
- Healthy Fats: 8g

Directions:

1. In a large pot, brown ground turkey until fully cooked.
2. Add carrots, celery, onion, and garlic. Sauté until vegetables are softened.
3. Pour in chicken broth, add lentils, thyme, salt, and pepper. Simmer for 30 minutes or until lentils are tender.
4. Serve hot.

Serving Methods:

- Sprinkle with chopped fresh parsley.
- Enjoy with a slice of whole-grain bread.

Mediterranean Chickpea Wraps

A delightful and Mediterranean-inspired wrap featuring chickpeas, tomatoes, cucumbers, and feta, offering a refreshing and protein-rich lunch.

Ingredients:

- 1 can (15 oz) chickpeas, drained and rinsed
- 1 cup cherry tomatoes, halved
- 1/2 cucumber, diced
- 1/4 cup red onion, finely chopped
- 2 tablespoons feta cheese, crumbled

- 2 whole-grain wraps

Prep Time: 15 minutes

Serving Size: 2

Serving Time: Lunch

Nutritional Information (per serving):

- Calories: 330
- Protein: 15g
- Fiber: 10g
- Healthy Fats: 10g

Directions:

1. In a bowl, combine chickpeas, cherry tomatoes, cucumber, red onion, and feta cheese.
2. Warm the whole-grain wraps.
3. Divide the chickpea mixture between the wraps.
4. Roll up and secure with toothpicks if needed.

Serving Methods:

- Drizzle with tzatziki sauce.
- Serve with a side of mixed greens.

Chicken and Avocado Lettuce Wraps

A light and protein-packed lunch option featuring seasoned chicken and creamy avocado wrapped in fresh lettuce leaves for a satisfying and low-carb meal.

Ingredients:

- 8 oz chicken breast, cooked and shredded
- 2 large iceberg lettuce leaves
- 1 avocado, sliced
- 1/2 cup cherry tomatoes, halved
- 1/4 cup red onion, thinly sliced
- 1 tablespoon cilantro, chopped

- Juice of 1 lime
- Salt and pepper to taste

Prep Time: 15 minutes

Cooking Time: 15 minutes (for chicken)

Serving Size: 2 wraps

Serving Time: Lunch

Nutritional Information (per serving):

- Calories: 300
- Protein: 20g
- Fiber: 8g
- Healthy Fats: 15g

Directions:

1. Season chicken breast with salt and pepper, then grill or sauté until fully cooked. Shred the cooked chicken.
2. In each lettuce leaf, layer shredded chicken, avocado slices, cherry tomatoes, red onion, and cilantro.
3. Squeeze lime juice over the fillings.
4. Roll up the lettuce leaves and secure with toothpicks if needed.

Serving Methods:

1. Drizzle with a light vinaigrette.
2. Serve with a side of salsa for added flavor.

Baked Salmon with Lemon Dill Sauce

A simple and elegant baked salmon dish with a zesty lemon dill sauce, providing omega-3 fatty acids and a burst of flavor for a wholesome lunch.

Ingredients:

- 6 oz salmon fillet
- 1 tablespoon olive oil
- 1 teaspoon lemon zest

- 1 tablespoon fresh dill, chopped
- Salt and pepper to taste

Prep Time: 10 minutes

Cooking Time: 20 minutes

Serving Size: 1

Serving Time: Lunch

Nutritional Information (per serving):

- Calories: 300
- Protein: 25g
- Fiber: 1g
- Healthy Fats: 20g

Directions:

1. Preheat the oven to 375°F (190°C).
2. Place the salmon fillet on a baking sheet.
3. Drizzle with olive oil, sprinkle lemon zest, fresh dill, salt, and pepper.
4. Bake for 20 minutes or until the salmon flakes easily with a fork.

Serving Methods:

- Serve over a bed of sautéed spinach.
- Drizzle with extra lemon dill sauce.

Quinoa and Black Bean Stuffed Peppers

A protein-packed and fiber-rich dish where bell peppers are filled with a mixture of quinoa, black beans, and spices, creating a nutritious and satisfying lunch.

Ingredients: 2 bell peppers, halved and seeds removed

- 1/2 cup cooked quinoa
- 1/2 cup black beans, drained and rinsed
- 1/4 cup corn kernels
- 1/4 cup red onion, finely chopped

- 1 teaspoon cumin
- 1/2 teaspoon chili powder
- Salt and pepper to taste

Prep Time: 20 minutes

Cooking Time: 25 minutes (includes baking time)

Serving Size: 2 halves

Serving Time: Lunch

Nutritional Information (per serving):

- Calories: 300
- Protein: 15g
- Fiber: 8g
- Healthy Fats: 5g

Directions:

1. Preheat the oven to 375°F (190°C).
2. In a bowl, mix together cooked quinoa, black beans, corn, red onion, cumin, chili powder, salt, and pepper.
3. Stuff the bell pepper halves with the quinoa and black bean mixture.
4. Bake for 25 minutes or until peppers are tender.

Serving Methods:

- Top with a dollop of Greek yogurt.
- Serve with a side of salsa for added flavor.

Turkey and Vegetable Skewers

A colorful and protein-rich dish featuring turkey and a variety of vegetables, grilled to perfection and served on skewers for a visually appealing and tasty lunch.

Ingredients: 8 oz turkey breast, cut into cubes

- 1/2 zucchini, sliced
- 1/2 red bell pepper, diced

- 1/2 yellow bell pepper, diced
- 1/2 red onion, cut into wedges
- 1 tablespoon olive oil
- 1 teaspoon dried oregano
- Salt and pepper to taste

Prep Time: 20 minutes

Cooking Time: 15 minutes

Serving Size: 1

Serving Time: Lunch

Nutritional Information (per serving):

- Calories: 320
- Protein: 25g
- Fiber: 6g
- Healthy Fats: 10g

Directions:

1. Preheat the grill or grill pan.
2. In a bowl, toss turkey cubes, zucchini, red bell pepper, yellow bell pepper, and red onion with olive oil, dried oregano, salt, and pepper.
3. Thread the turkey and vegetable pieces onto skewers.
4. Grill for 15 minutes or until turkey is cooked through.

Serving Methods:

- Serve over a bed of quinoa.
- Drizzle with a balsamic glaze for added flavor.

Eggplant and Chickpea Curry

A flavorful and plant-based curry featuring eggplant, chickpeas, and aromatic spices, offering a hearty and satisfying lunch option.

Ingredients: 1 large eggplant, cubed

- 1 can (15 oz) chickpeas, drained and rinsed

- 1 cup tomatoes, diced
- 1 onion, finely chopped
- 2 cloves garlic, minced
- 1 tablespoon curry powder
- 1 teaspoon cumin
- 1 teaspoon turmeric
- 1/2 teaspoon chili powder
- 1 cup vegetable broth
- 2 tablespoons coconut milk
- Fresh cilantro for garnish

Prep Time: 20 minutes

Cooking Time: 25 minutes

Serving Size: 1

Serving Time: Lunch

Nutritional Information (per serving):

- Calories: 350
- Protein: 15g
- Fiber: 10g
- Healthy Fats: 8g

Directions:

1. In a pot, sauté onions and garlic until softened.
2. Add eggplant, chickpeas, tomatoes, curry powder, cumin, turmeric, and chili powder. Stir to coat.
3. Pour in vegetable broth and coconut milk. Simmer for 25 minutes or until eggplant is tender.
4. Garnish with fresh cilantro before serving.

Serving Methods:

- Serve over brown rice.
- Enjoy with a side of whole-grain naan.

Spinach and Mushroom Omelette

A nutrient-packed omelette featuring spinach, mushrooms, and cheese, offering a quick and protein-rich lunch option.

Ingredients:

- 2 large eggs, beaten
- 1 cup fresh spinach leaves
- 1/2 cup mushrooms, sliced
- 1/4 cup shredded cheese (cheddar or feta)
- 1 tablespoon olive oil
- Salt and pepper to taste

Prep Time: 10 minutes

Cooking Time: 5 minutes

Serving Size: 1

Serving Time: Lunch

Nutritional Information (per serving):

- Calories: 280
- Protein: 15g
- Fiber: 3g
- Healthy Fats: 20g

Directions:

1. In a non-stick skillet, heat olive oil over medium heat.
2. Sauté mushrooms until browned.
3. Add fresh spinach and cook until wilted.
4. Pour beaten eggs over the vegetables, sprinkle with cheese, and cook until set.

Serving Methods:

- Fold in half and serve on whole-grain toast.
- Garnish with diced tomatoes and avocado.

Tofu and Vegetable Skillet

A plant-based and protein-rich skillet featuring tofu, assorted vegetables, and a flavorful sauce, providing a delicious and balanced lunch.

Ingredients:

- 8 oz firm tofu, cubed
- 1 cup broccoli florets
- 1/2 cup bell peppers, sliced
- 1/2 cup snow peas
- 1/4 cup soy sauce
- 1 tablespoon sesame oil
- 1 tablespoon rice vinegar
- 1 tablespoon maple syrup
- 1 teaspoon ginger, minced
- 1 clove garlic, minced

Prep Time: 15 minutes

Cooking Time: 15 minutes

Serving Size: 1

Serving Time: Lunch

Nutritional Information (per serving):

- Calories: 310
- Protein: 20g
- Fiber: 8g
- Healthy Fats: 15g

Directions:

1. Press tofu to remove excess moisture, then cube it.
2. In a skillet, sauté tofu until golden brown.
3. Add broccoli, bell peppers, and snow peas. Stir-fry until vegetables are tender-crisp.

4. In a small bowl, whisk together soy sauce, sesame oil, rice vinegar, maple syrup, ginger, and garlic. Pour over the tofu and vegetables, stirring to coat.

Serving Methods:

- Serve over a bed of brown rice or quinoa.
- Garnish with sliced green onions.

DINNER RECIPES

Grilled Salmon with Lemon-Dill Sauce

A heart-healthy dinner featuring grilled salmon fillets topped with a zesty lemon-dill sauce, providing omega-3 fatty acids and fresh flavors.

Ingredients:

- 2 salmon fillets (6 oz each)
- 1 tablespoon olive oil
- 1 teaspoon lemon zest
- 1 tablespoon fresh dill, chopped
- Salt and pepper to taste

Prep Time: 10 minutes

Cooking Time: 15 minutes

Serving Size: 1

Serving Time: Dinner

Nutritional Information (per serving):

- Calories: 300
- Protein: 25g
- Fiber: 1g
- Healthy Fats: 20g

Directions:

1. Preheat the grill to medium-high heat.
2. Brush salmon fillets with olive oil and season with salt, pepper, lemon zest, and fresh dill.
3. Grill for 6-8 minutes per side or until salmon flakes easily with a fork.
4. Serve with a side of steamed vegetables or quinoa.

Serving Methods:

- Drizzle with additional lemon-dill sauce.

- Garnish with a wedge of lemon for extra freshness.

Mediterranean Chicken Skewers

A delightful and protein-packed dinner option featuring marinated chicken skewers with Mediterranean flavors, served with a refreshing cucumber salad.

Ingredients:

- 8 oz chicken breast, cut into cubes
- 1 tablespoon olive oil
- 1 teaspoon dried oregano
- 1 teaspoon paprika
- 1/2 teaspoon garlic powder
- Salt and pepper to taste

Cucumber Salad:

- 1 cucumber, diced
- 1 cup cherry tomatoes, halved
- 1/4 cup red onion, finely chopped
- Feta cheese for garnish

Prep Time: 20 minutes

Cooking Time: 10 minutes

Serving Size: 1

Serving Time: Dinner

Nutritional Information (per serving):

- Calories: 350
- Protein: 30g
- Fiber: 4g
- Healthy Fats: 15g

Directions:

1. In a bowl, mix olive oil, dried oregano, paprika, garlic powder, salt, and pepper. Marinate chicken cubes for 15 minutes.

2. Thread marinated chicken onto skewers and grill for 5 minutes per side or until cooked through.
3. In a separate bowl, combine cucumber, cherry tomatoes, and red onion for the salad.
4. Serve chicken skewers over a bed of cucumber salad and sprinkle with feta.

Serving Methods:

- Drizzle with a balsamic glaze.
- Serve with a side of whole-grain couscous.

Quinoa and Vegetable Stuffed Bell Peppers

A nutrient-packed dinner where bell peppers are filled with a mixture of quinoa, vegetables, and lean ground turkey, creating a wholesome and balanced meal.

Ingredients: 2 bell peppers, halved and seeds removed

- 1/2 cup cooked quinoa
- 8 oz lean ground turkey
- 1/2 cup black beans, drained and rinsed
- 1/4 cup corn kernels
- 1/4 cup red onion, finely chopped
- 1 teaspoon cumin
- 1/2 teaspoon chili powder
- Salt and pepper to taste

Prep Time: 20 minutes

Cooking Time: 25 minutes (includes baking time)

Serving Size: 2 halves

Serving Time: Dinner

Nutritional Information (per serving):

- Calories: 350
- Protein: 25g

- Fiber: 8g
- Healthy Fats: 10g

Directions:

1. Preheat the oven to 375°F (190°C).
2. In a bowl, mix together cooked quinoa, ground turkey, black beans, corn, red onion, cumin, chili powder, salt, and pepper.
3. Stuff the bell pepper halves with the quinoa and turkey mixture.
4. Bake for 25 minutes or until peppers are tender.
5. Serve with a side of salsa or guacamole.

Serving Methods:

- Top with a dollop of Greek yogurt.
- Serve with a side of mixed greens.

Baked Chicken with Rosemary and Lemon

A simple and flavorful baked chicken dish with the aromatic combination of rosemary and lemon, offering a light and satisfying dinner.

Ingredients:

- 2 chicken breasts (6 oz each)
- 1 tablespoon olive oil
- 1 tablespoon fresh rosemary, chopped
- 1 lemon, sliced
- Salt and pepper to taste

Prep Time: 10 minutes

Cooking Time: 25 minutes

Serving Size: 1

Serving Time: Dinner

Nutritional Information (per serving):

- Calories: 320
- Protein: 30g
- Fiber: 1g

- Healthy Fats: 15g

Directions:

1. Preheat the oven to 375°F (190°C).
2. Rub chicken breasts with olive oil, chopped rosemary, salt, and pepper.
3. Place lemon slices on top of the chicken.
4. Bake for 25 minutes or until chicken is cooked through.
5. Serve with a side of steamed vegetables or roasted sweet potatoes.

Serving Methods:

- Drizzle with extra olive oil.
- Garnish with additional fresh rosemary.

Shrimp and Asparagus Stir-Fry

A quick and low-calorie dinner option featuring succulent shrimp, crisp asparagus, and a flavorful stir-fry sauce, providing a balanced and tasty meal.

Ingredients:

- 8 oz shrimp, peeled and deveined
- 1 bunch asparagus, trimmed and cut into bite-sized pieces
- 1 tablespoon sesame oil
- 2 tablespoons low-sodium soy sauce
- 1 tablespoon rice vinegar
- 1 teaspoon honey
- 1 teaspoon ginger, minced
- 2 cloves garlic, minced

Prep Time: 15 minutes

Cooking Time: 10 minutes

Serving Size: 1

Serving Time: Dinner

Nutritional Information (per serving):

- Calories: 280
- Protein: 20g
- Fiber: 5g
- Healthy Fats: 10g

Directions:

1. In a wok or skillet, heat sesame oil and sauté garlic and ginger until fragrant.
2. Add shrimp and cook until pink and opaque.
3. Add asparagus and stir-fry for an additional 3-4 minutes.
4. In a small bowl, mix soy sauce, rice vinegar, and honey. Pour over the shrimp and asparagus.
5. Serve over a bed of brown rice or cauliflower rice.

Serving Methods:

- Garnish with sesame seeds.
- Drizzle with sriracha for extra heat.

Lentil and Vegetable Curry

A comforting and fiber-rich lentil and vegetable curry with aromatic spices, providing a vegetarian dinner option that's both nutritious and satisfying.

Ingredients:

- 1 cup dry lentils, rinsed and drained
- 2 cups vegetable broth
- 1 cup sweet potatoes, diced
- 1 cup cauliflower florets
- 1 cup cherry tomatoes, halved
- 1 onion, finely chopped
- 2 cloves garlic, minced
- 1 tablespoon curry powder
- 1 teaspoon cumin
- 1/2 teaspoon turmeric
- Salt and pepper to taste

Prep Time: 20 minutes

Cooking Time: 30 minutes

Serving Size: 2

Serving Time: Dinner

Nutritional Information (per serving):

- Calories: 320
- Protein: 18g
- Fiber: 12g
- Healthy Fats: 5g

Directions:

1. In a large pot, sauté onions and garlic until softened.
2. Add lentils, vegetable broth, sweet potatoes, cauliflower, cherry tomatoes, curry powder, cumin, turmeric, salt, and pepper.
3. Simmer for 30 minutes or until lentils and vegetables are tender.
4. Serve over a bed of brown rice.

Serving Methods:

- Garnish with fresh cilantro.
- Enjoy with a side of whole-grain naan.

Turkey and Vegetable Stir-Fry

A quick and savory turkey and vegetable stir-fry with a flavorful sauce, offering a protein-packed and low-carb dinner option.

Ingredients: 8 oz lean ground turkey

- 1 cup broccoli florets
- 1/2 cup bell peppers, sliced
- 1/2 cup snap peas, halved
- 1/4 cup carrots, julienned
- 2 tablespoons low-sodium soy sauce
- 1 tablespoon hoisin sauce
- 1 teaspoon sesame oil

- 1 teaspoon ginger, minced
- 2 cloves garlic, minced

Prep Time: 15 minutes

Cooking Time: 10 minutes

Serving Size: 1

Serving Time: Dinner

Nutritional Information (per serving):

- Calories: 320
- Protein: 25g
- Fiber: 6g
- Healthy Fats: 12g

Directions:

1. In a wok or skillet, brown ground turkey until fully cooked.
2. Add broccoli, bell peppers, snap peas, and carrots. Stir-fry until vegetables are tender-crisp.
3. In a small bowl, whisk together soy sauce, hoisin sauce, sesame oil, ginger, and garlic. Pour over the turkey and vegetables.
4. Serve over cauliflower rice or quinoa.

Serving Methods:

- Top with sliced green onions.
- Sprinkle with sesame seeds for added texture.

Chickpea and Spinach Stew

A hearty and nutritious chickpea and spinach stew with warming spices, creating a flavorful and plant-based dinner option.

Ingredients: 1 can (15 oz) chickpeas, drained and rinsed

- 2 cups fresh spinach leaves
- 1 cup tomatoes, diced
- 1 onion, finely chopped
- 2 cloves garlic, minced

- 1 teaspoon cumin
- 1/2 teaspoon paprika
- 1/4 teaspoon cayenne pepper
- 2 cups vegetable broth
- 1 tablespoon olive oil

Prep Time: 15 minutes

Cooking Time: 25 minutes

Serving Size: 2

Serving Time: Dinner

Nutritional Information (per serving):

- Calories: 300
- Protein: 14g
- Fiber: 10g
- Healthy Fats: 10g

Directions:

1. In a pot, sauté onions and garlic in olive oil until softened.
2. Add chickpeas, spinach, tomatoes, cumin, paprika, cayenne pepper, and vegetable broth.
3. Simmer for 25 minutes or until flavors meld and stew thickens.
4. Serve with a side of whole-grain bread or brown rice.

Serving Methods:

- Garnish with a dollop of Greek yogurt.
- Sprinkle with chopped fresh parsley.

Vegetable and Tofu Stir-Fry

A colorful and plant-based stir-fry featuring tofu and a variety of vegetables, tossed in a savory sauce, providing a nutritious and satisfying dinner.

Ingredients: 8 oz firm tofu, cubed

- 1 cup broccoli florets

- 1/2 cup bell peppers, sliced
- 1/2 cup snow peas
- 1/4 cup carrots, julienned
- 2 tablespoons low-sodium soy sauce
- 1 tablespoon hoisin sauce
- 1 tablespoon sesame oil
- 1 teaspoon ginger, minced
- 2 cloves garlic, minced

Prep Time: 20 minutes

Cooking Time: 15 minutes

Serving Size: 1

Serving Time: Dinner

Nutritional Information (per serving):

- Calories: 310
- Protein: 20g
- Fiber: 8g
- Healthy Fats: 15g

Directions:

1. Press tofu to remove excess moisture, then cube it.
2. In a wok or skillet, heat sesame oil and sauté garlic and ginger until fragrant.
3. Add tofu, broccoli, bell peppers, snow peas, and carrots. Stir-fry until tofu is golden and vegetables are tender-crisp.
4. In a small bowl, whisk together soy sauce and hoisin sauce. Pour over the tofu and vegetables.
5. Serve over a bed of brown rice or cauliflower rice.

Serving Methods:

- Garnish with sesame seeds.
- Drizzle with sriracha for added heat.

Baked Eggplant Parmesan

A lighter and healthier version of the classic Eggplant Parmesan, featuring baked eggplant slices, marinara sauce, and melted cheese for a satisfying and flavorful dinner.

Ingredients:

- 1 large eggplant, sliced
- 1 cup whole-grain breadcrumbs
- 1/2 cup grated Parmesan cheese
- 2 cups marinara sauce
- 1 cup part-skim mozzarella cheese, shredded
- Fresh basil for garnish

Prep Time: 20 minutes

Cooking Time: 25 minutes

Serving Size: 2

Serving Time: Dinner

Nutritional Information (per serving):

- Calories: 320
- Protein: 15g
- Fiber: 10g
- Healthy Fats: 10g

Directions:

1. Preheat the oven to 375°F (190°C).
2. Dip eggplant slices in whole-grain breadcrumbs and arrange on a baking sheet.
3. Bake for 15 minutes, flipping halfway through, until golden brown.
4. In a baking dish, layer baked eggplant slices, marinara sauce, and Parmesan cheese. Repeat layers.

5. Top with shredded mozzarella and bake for an additional 10 minutes or until cheese is melted.
6. Garnish with fresh basil before serving.

Serving Methods:

1. Serve over a bed of whole-grain pasta.
2. Pair with a side salad for added freshness.

Lemon Garlic Herb Baked Chicken

A flavorful and herb-infused baked chicken dish with a zesty lemon and garlic marinade, providing a light yet satisfying dinner.

Ingredients:

- 2 chicken breasts (6 oz each)
- 2 tablespoons olive oil
- 1 tablespoon fresh herbs (rosemary, thyme, or oregano)
- Zest of 1 lemon
- 2 cloves garlic, minced
- Salt and pepper to taste

Prep Time: 15 minutes

Cooking Time: 25 minutes

Serving Size: 1

Serving Time: Dinner

Nutritional Information (per serving):

- Calories: 320
- Protein: 30g
- Fiber: 1g
- Healthy Fats: 15g

Directions:

1. Preheat the oven to 375°F (190°C).
2. Mix olive oil, fresh herbs, lemon zest, minced garlic, salt, and pepper to create a marinade.

3. Rub the chicken breasts with the marinade and let them sit for 15 minutes.
4. Bake for 25 minutes or until chicken is cooked through.
5. Serve with a side of roasted vegetables or quinoa.

Serving Methods:

- Drizzle with extra lemon juice.
- Garnish with chopped fresh herbs.

Lentil and Vegetable Stir-Fry

A quick and nutritious stir-fry featuring protein-packed lentils and a colorful array of vegetables, creating a satisfying and plant-based dinner.

Ingredients:

- 1 cup dry lentils, cooked
- 1 cup broccoli florets
- 1/2 cup bell peppers, sliced
- 1/2 cup snap peas, halved
- 1/4 cup carrots, julienned
- 2 tablespoons low-sodium soy sauce
- 1 tablespoon sesame oil
- 1 teaspoon ginger, minced
- 2 cloves garlic, minced

Prep Time: 20 minutes

Cooking Time: 10 minutes

Serving Size: 1

Serving Time: Dinner

Nutritional Information (per serving):

- Calories: 340
- Protein: 20g
- Fiber: 12g
- Healthy Fats: 8g

Directions:

1. Cook lentils according to package instructions.
2. In a wok or skillet, heat sesame oil and sauté garlic and ginger until fragrant.
3. Add cooked lentils, broccoli, bell peppers, snap peas, and carrots. Stir-fry until vegetables are tender-crisp.
4. Stir in low-sodium soy sauce.
5. Serve over brown rice or cauliflower rice.

Serving Methods:

- Top with a sprinkle of sesame seeds.
- Drizzle with a touch of teriyaki sauce.

Mediterranean Turkey Burgers

A lean and flavorful dinner option featuring turkey burgers seasoned with Mediterranean herbs and served with a refreshing cucumber and tomato salad.

Ingredients:

- 8 oz ground turkey
- 1/4 cup feta cheese, crumbled
- 1 teaspoon dried oregano
- 1/2 teaspoon garlic powder
- Salt and pepper to taste

Cucumber and Tomato Salad:

- 1 cucumber, diced
- 1 cup cherry tomatoes, halved
- 2 tablespoons red onion, finely chopped
- Fresh mint for garnish

Prep Time: 15 minutes

Cooking Time: 15 minutes

Serving Size: 2

Serving Time: Dinner

Nutritional Information (per serving):

- Calories: 320
- Protein: 25g
- Fiber: 3g
- Healthy Fats: 15g

Directions:

1. In a bowl, mix ground turkey, feta cheese, dried oregano, garlic powder, salt, and pepper. Form into patties.
2. Grill or pan-sear the turkey burgers for 6-8 minutes per side.
3. In a separate bowl, combine diced cucumber, cherry tomatoes, and red onion for the salad.
4. Serve turkey burgers on a whole-grain bun or lettuce wrap with a side of cucumber and tomato salad.

Serving Methods:

- Drizzle with a tzatziki sauce.
- Garnish with fresh mint leaves.

Teriyaki Salmon with Stir-Fried Vegetables

A savory and sweet teriyaki-glazed salmon served with a medley of stir-fried vegetables, creating a balanced and flavorful dinner.

Ingredients:

- 2 salmon fillets (6 oz each)
- 2 tablespoons low-sodium teriyaki sauce
- 1 tablespoon olive oil
- 1 cup broccoli florets
- 1/2 cup bell peppers, sliced
- 1/2 cup snow peas
- 1/4 cup carrots, julienned
- 1 teaspoon sesame seeds for garnish

Prep Time: 15 minutes

Cooking Time: 15 minutes

Serving Size: 1

Serving Time: Dinner

Nutritional Information (per serving):

- Calories: 350
- Protein: 30g
- Fiber: 6g
- Healthy Fats: 18g

Directions:

1. Preheat the oven to 375°F (190°C).
2. Place salmon fillets on a baking sheet, brush with teriyaki sauce, and bake for 15 minutes or until salmon flakes easily with a fork.
3. In a skillet, heat olive oil and stir-fry broccoli, bell peppers, snow peas, and carrots until tender-crisp.
4. Serve teriyaki salmon over the stir-fried vegetables.
5. Sprinkle with sesame seeds.

Serving Methods:

- Serve over a bed of quinoa.
- Drizzle with extra teriyaki sauce.

Cauliflower and Chickpea Curry

A comforting and plant-based curry featuring cauliflower and chickpeas in a flavorful coconut milk base, providing a rich and satisfying dinner.

Ingredients:

- 1/2 head cauliflower, cut into florets
- 1 can (15 oz) chickpeas, drained and rinsed
- 1 cup tomatoes, diced
- 1 onion, finely chopped
- 2 cloves garlic, minced
- 1 tablespoon curry powder

- 1 teaspoon cumin
- 1/2 teaspoon turmeric
- 1 cup coconut milk
- Fresh cilantro for garnish

Prep Time: 20 minutes

Cooking Time: 25 minutes

Serving Size: 2

Serving Time: Dinner

Nutritional Information (per serving):

- Calories: 320
- Protein: 14g
- Fiber: 10g
- Healthy Fats: 10g

Directions:

1. In a pot, sauté onions and garlic until softened.
2. Add cauliflower, chickpeas, tomatoes, curry powder, cumin, turmeric, and coconut milk. Stir to combine.
3. Simmer for 25 minutes or until cauliflower is tender.
4. Garnish with fresh cilantro before serving.
5. Serve over a bed of brown rice.

Serving Methods:

- Enjoy with a side of naan bread.
- Sprinkle with a dash of lime juice.

Balsamic Glazed Chicken with Roasted Vegetables

A sweet and tangy balsamic-glazed chicken accompanied by a medley of roasted vegetables, creating a delicious and well-balanced dinner.

Ingredients:

- 2 chicken breasts (6 oz each)
- 2 tablespoons balsamic glaze

- 1 tablespoon olive oil
- 1 cup baby potatoes, halved
- 1 cup carrots, sliced
- 1 cup Brussels sprouts, halved
- Salt and pepper to taste

Prep Time: 20 minutes

Cooking Time: 30 minutes

Serving Size: 1

Serving Time: Dinner

Nutritional Information (per serving):

- Calories: 340
- Protein: 28g
- Fiber: 6g
- Healthy Fats: 15g

Directions:

1. Preheat the oven to 400°F (200°C).
2. Place chicken breasts on a baking sheet, brush with balsamic glaze, and season with salt and pepper.
3. In a bowl, toss baby potatoes, carrots, and Brussels sprouts with olive oil, salt, and pepper.
4. Arrange vegetables around the chicken on the baking sheet.
5. Roast for 30 minutes or until chicken is cooked through and vegetables are tender.
6. Serve with a side of quinoa or brown rice.

Serving Methods:

- Drizzle with additional balsamic glaze.
- Garnish with fresh parsley.

Spaghetti Squash with Turkey Bolognese

A low-carb alternative to traditional pasta, featuring spaghetti squash topped with a lean turkey Bolognese sauce for a wholesome and satisfying dinner.

Ingredients:

- 1 spaghetti squash, halved and seeds removed
- 8 oz lean ground turkey
- 1 cup tomatoes, crushed
- 1/2 cup carrots, finely chopped
- 1/4 cup celery, finely chopped
- 2 cloves garlic, minced
- 1 teaspoon dried oregano
- 1/2 teaspoon red pepper flakes (optional)
- Salt and pepper to taste

Prep Time: 15 minutes

Cooking Time: 45 minutes

Serving Size: 2

Serving Time: Dinner

Nutritional Information (per serving):

- Calories: 300
- Protein: 22g
- Fiber: 8g
- Healthy Fats: 10g

Directions:

1. Preheat the oven to 400°F (200°C).
2. Place spaghetti squash halves on a baking sheet, cut side down, and roast for 40 minutes or until tender.

3. In a skillet, brown ground turkey. Add garlic, carrots, celery, dried oregano, red pepper flakes (if using), salt, and pepper.
4. Stir in crushed tomatoes and simmer for 15 minutes.
5. Scrape the flesh of the cooked spaghetti squash with a fork to create "noodles" and top with turkey Bolognese.

Serving Methods:

*   Sprinkle with grated Parmesan cheese.
*   Garnish with fresh basil.

Seared Tofu with Quinoa and Broccoli

A protein-packed vegetarian dinner featuring seared tofu served over a bed of quinoa with steamed broccoli, creating a well-balanced and nutritious meal.

Ingredients:

*   8 oz firm tofu, sliced
*   1 cup cooked quinoa
*   1 cup broccoli florets
*   2 tablespoons soy sauce
*   1 tablespoon sesame oil
*   1 teaspoon ginger, minced
*   2 cloves garlic, minced

Prep Time: 20 minutes

Cooking Time: 15 minutes

Serving Size: 1

Serving Time: Dinner

Nutritional Information (per serving):

*   Calories: 330
*   Protein: 20g
*   Fiber: 6g
*   Healthy Fats: 15g

Directions:

1. Press tofu to remove excess moisture, then sear in a non-stick skillet until golden brown on both sides.
2. In the same skillet, sauté garlic and ginger until fragrant.
3. Add cooked quinoa and broccoli florets. Stir in soy sauce and sesame oil.
4. Serve seared tofu over the quinoa and broccoli mixture.

Serving Methods:

- Drizzle with extra soy sauce.
- Top with sliced green onions.

Stuffed Bell Peppers with Quinoa and Black Beans

A colorful and fiber-rich dinner featuring bell peppers stuffed with a mixture of quinoa, black beans, and savory spices, providing a wholesome and satisfying meal.

Ingredients:

- 2 bell peppers, halved and seeds removed
- 1/2 cup cooked quinoa
- 1/2 cup black beans, drained and rinsed
- 1/4 cup corn kernels
- 1/4 cup red onion, finely chopped
- 1 teaspoon cumin
- 1/2 teaspoon chili powder
- Salt and pepper to taste

Prep Time: 20 minutes

Cooking Time: 25 minutes (includes baking time)

Serving Size: 2 halves

Serving Time: Dinner

Nutritional Information (per serving):

- Calories: 350
- Protein: 25g
- Fiber: 8g
- Healthy Fats: 10g

Directions:

1. Preheat the oven to 375°F (190°C).
2. In a bowl, mix together cooked quinoa, black beans, corn, red onion, cumin, chili powder, salt, and pepper.
3. Stuff the bell pepper halves with the quinoa and black bean mixture.
4. Bake for 25 minutes or until peppers are tender.
5. Serve with a side of salsa or guacamole.

Serving Methods:

- Top with a dollop of Greek yogurt.
- Serve with a side of mixed greens.

Shrimp and Vegetable Skewers

A delightful and protein-rich dinner featuring grilled shrimp skewers with a colorful array of vegetables, served with a refreshing citrus dipping sauce.

Ingredients:

- 8 oz shrimp, peeled and deveined
- 1 bell pepper, cut into chunks
- 1 zucchini, sliced
- 1 cup cherry tomatoes
- 1 tablespoon olive oil
- 1 teaspoon lemon zest
- 1 tablespoon fresh parsley, chopped
- Salt and pepper to taste

Prep Time: 20 minutes

Cooking Time: 10 minutes

Serving Size: 1

Serving Time: Dinner

Nutritional Information (per serving):

- Calories: 280
- Protein: 20g
- Fiber: 4g
- Healthy Fats: 10g

Directions:

1. Preheat the grill to medium-high heat.
2. Thread shrimp, bell pepper chunks, zucchini slices, and cherry tomatoes onto skewers.
3. Mix olive oil, lemon zest, chopped parsley, salt, and pepper to create a marinade.
4. Brush skewers with the marinade and grill for 4-5 minutes per side or until shrimp are opaque.
5. Serve with a side of quinoa or couscous.

Serving Methods:

- Drizzle with additional citrus sauce.
- Garnish with extra fresh parsley.

SIDE DISHES

Quinoa and Vegetable Pilaf

A nutritious and fiber-rich side dish featuring quinoa mixed with colorful vegetables, creating a wholesome accompaniment to any meal.

Ingredients: 1 cup quinoa, rinsed

- 2 cups vegetable broth
- 1 cup mixed vegetables (carrots, peas, corn)
- 1/4 cup red onion, finely chopped
- 2 tablespoons olive oil
- Salt and pepper to taste

Prep Time: 15 minutes

Cooking Time: 20 minutes

Serving Size: 1/2 cup

Serving Time: Lunch or Dinner

Nutritional Information (per serving):

- Calories: 180
- Protein: 5g
- Fiber: 4g
- Healthy Fats: 7g

Directions:

1. In a pot, sauté red onion in olive oil until softened.
2. Add quinoa and stir for 1-2 minutes.
3. Pour in vegetable broth and bring to a boil. Reduce heat, cover, and simmer for 15-20 minutes or until quinoa is cooked.
4. In the last 5 minutes of cooking, add mixed vegetables.
5. Fluff with a fork and season with salt and pepper.

Serving Methods:

- Sprinkle with fresh herbs (parsley or cilantro).

- Serve alongside grilled chicken or fish.

Roasted Brussels Sprouts with Balsamic Glaze

A flavorful side dish featuring roasted Brussels sprouts drizzled with a sweet and tangy balsamic glaze, adding a delightful twist to a classic vegetable.

Ingredients:

- 1 lb Brussels sprouts, halved
- 2 tablespoons olive oil
- 2 tablespoons balsamic glaze
- Salt and pepper to taste

Prep Time: 10 minutes

Cooking Time: 25 minutes

Serving Size: 1/2 cup

Serving Time: Dinner

Nutritional Information (per serving):

- Calories: 90
- Protein: 3g
- Fiber: 4g
- Healthy Fats: 5g

Directions:

1. Preheat the oven to 400°F (200°C).
2. Toss Brussels sprouts with olive oil, salt, and pepper.
3. Roast for 20-25 minutes or until golden and crispy.
4. Drizzle with balsamic glaze before serving.

Serving Methods:

- Sprinkle with grated Parmesan cheese.
- Garnish with toasted pine nuts.

Garlic and Herb Cauliflower Mash

A low-carb alternative to traditional mashed potatoes, featuring cauliflower blended with garlic and herbs for a creamy and flavorful side.

Ingredients:

- 1 head cauliflower, cut into florets
- 2 cloves garlic, minced
- 2 tablespoons unsalted butter
- 1/4 cup low-fat milk
- Fresh herbs (parsley or chives)
- Salt and pepper to taste

Prep Time: 15 minutes

Cooking Time: 15 minutes

Serving Size: 1/2 cup

Serving Time: Dinner

Nutritional Information (per serving):

- Calories: 70
- Protein: 3g
- Fiber: 4g
- Healthy Fats: 4g

Directions:

1. Steam or boil cauliflower until tender.
2. In a blender, combine cauliflower, minced garlic, butter, and milk. Blend until smooth.
3. Season with salt and pepper, and stir in fresh herbs before serving.

Serving Methods:

- Top with a dollop of Greek yogurt.
- Serve alongside roasted chicken or grilled fish.

Spinach and Mushroom Salad with Lemon Vinaigrette

A refreshing and nutrient-packed salad featuring fresh spinach, mushrooms, and a zesty lemon vinaigrette for a light and vibrant side.

Ingredients:

- 4 cups fresh spinach leaves
- 1 cup mushrooms, sliced
- 1/4 cup red onion, thinly sliced
- 1 tablespoon olive oil
- Juice of 1 lemon
- Salt and pepper to taste

Prep Time: 10 minutes

Cooking Time: 0 minutes

Serving Size: 1 cup

Serving Time: Lunch or Dinner

Nutritional Information (per serving):

- Calories: 80
- Protein: 3g
- Fiber: 3g
- Healthy Fats: 6g

Directions:

1. In a large bowl, combine fresh spinach, sliced mushrooms, and red onion.
2. In a small bowl, whisk together olive oil, lemon juice, salt, and pepper.
3. Toss the salad with the lemon vinaigrette just before serving.

Serving Methods:

- Top with crumbled feta cheese.
- Serve as a side with grilled shrimp or chicken.

Lemon Garlic Asparagus

A simple yet flavorful side dish featuring asparagus spears roasted with lemon and garlic, providing a bright and nutritious addition to any meal.

Ingredients:

- 1 lb asparagus, trimmed
- 2 tablespoons olive oil
- Zest of 1 lemon
- 2 cloves garlic, minced
- Salt and pepper to taste

Prep Time: 10 minutes

Cooking Time: 15 minutes

Serving Size: 1/2 cup

Serving Time: Dinner

Nutritional Information (per serving):

- Calories: 60
- Protein: 2g
- Fiber: 3g
- Healthy Fats: 5g

Directions:

1. Preheat the oven to 400°F (200°C).
2. Toss asparagus with olive oil, lemon zest, minced garlic, salt, and pepper.
3. Roast for 12-15 minutes or until asparagus is tender-crisp.

Serving Methods:

- Squeeze additional lemon juice before serving.
- Top with shaved Parmesan cheese.

Cucumber and Avocado Salad

A refreshing and creamy salad featuring cucumber and avocado, tossed with a light lemony dressing, creating a hydrating and nutrient-dense side.

Ingredients: 2 cucumbers, diced

- 2 avocados, diced
- 1/4 cup red onion, finely chopped
- 1 tablespoon fresh dill, chopped
- Juice of 1 lemon
- 1 tablespoon olive oil
- Salt and pepper to taste

Prep Time: 10 minutes

Cooking Time: 0 minutes

Serving Size: 1/2 cup

Serving Time: Lunch or Dinner

Nutritional Information (per serving):

- Calories: 120
- Protein: 2g
- Fiber: 6g
- Healthy Fats: 10g

Directions:

1. In a bowl, combine diced cucumbers, avocados, red onion, and fresh dill.
2. In a small bowl, whisk together lemon juice, olive oil, salt, and pepper.
3. Toss the salad with the dressing just before serving.

Serving Methods:

- Sprinkle with hemp seeds.
- Serve as a side with grilled chicken or fish.

Sweet Potato and Kale Hash

A nutrient-dense and colorful side dish featuring sweet potatoes and kale sautéed with aromatic spices, providing a delicious and hearty addition to any meal.

Ingredients:

- 2 sweet potatoes, peeled and diced
- 2 cups kale, chopped
- 1/4 cup red bell pepper, diced
- 1/4 cup red onion, finely chopped
- 1 tablespoon olive oil
- 1 teaspoon smoked paprika
- Salt and pepper to taste

Prep Time: 15 minutes

Cooking Time: 20 minutes

Serving Size: 1/2 cup

Serving Time: Breakfast or Lunch

Nutritional Information (per serving):

- Calories: 120
- Protein: 2g
- Fiber: 4g
- Healthy Fats: 5g

Directions:

1. In a skillet, heat olive oil and sauté red onion until softened.
2. Add diced sweet potatoes, smoked paprika, salt, and pepper. Cook until potatoes are golden brown.
3. Stir in chopped kale and red bell pepper. Cook until kale is wilted.

Serving Methods:

- Top with a poached egg for breakfast.
- Serve as a side with grilled salmon or tofu.

Greek Quinoa Salad

A Mediterranean-inspired side dish featuring quinoa, cherry tomatoes, cucumber, feta cheese, and olives, tossed in a lemony Greek dressing for a refreshing and nutritious salad.

Ingredients:

- 1 cup quinoa, cooked
- 1 cup cherry tomatoes, halved
- 1 cucumber, diced
- 1/2 cup feta cheese, crumbled
- 1/4 cup Kalamata olives, sliced
- Juice of 1 lemon
- 2 tablespoons olive oil
- Fresh oregano for garnish
- Salt and pepper to taste

Prep Time: 15 minutes

Cooking Time: 15 minutes (for quinoa)

Serving Size: 1/2 cup

Serving Time: Lunch or Dinner

Nutritional Information (per serving):

- Calories: 180
- Protein: 5g
- Fiber: 3g
- Healthy Fats: 10g

Directions:

1. In a large bowl, combine cooked quinoa, cherry tomatoes, cucumber, feta cheese, and Kalamata olives.
2. In a small bowl, whisk together lemon juice, olive oil, salt, and pepper.
3. Toss the salad with the dressing and garnish with fresh oregano.

Serving Methods:

- Top with grilled chicken or shrimp.
- Serve as a side with whole-grain pita.

Butternut Squash and Cranberry Quinoa

A festive and nutrient-dense side dish featuring butternut squash, quinoa, and cranberries, creating a flavorful and colorful addition to holiday meals.

Ingredients:

- 1 cup quinoa, cooked
- 1 cup butternut squash, diced
- 1/4 cup dried cranberries
- 2 tablespoons pecans, chopped
- 1 tablespoon maple syrup
- 1 tablespoon olive oil
- 1/2 teaspoon cinnamon
- Salt to taste

Prep Time: 15 minutes

Cooking Time: 20 minutes (for quinoa and squash)

Serving Size: 1/2 cup

Serving Time: Dinner

Nutritional Information (per serving):

- Calories: 160
- Protein: 4g
- Fiber: 3g
- Healthy Fats: 7g

Directions:

1. Roast diced butternut squash in the oven with olive oil, cinnamon, and salt until tender.

2. In a bowl, combine cooked quinoa, roasted butternut squash, dried cranberries, pecans, and maple syrup.
3. Toss gently to combine.

Serving Methods:

- Sprinkle with crumbled goat cheese.
- Serve as a side with roast turkey or chicken.

Grilled Eggplant with Tomato Salsa

A flavorful and antioxidant-rich side dish featuring grilled eggplant topped with a fresh tomato salsa, creating a delicious and vibrant addition to any meal.

Ingredients: 1 large eggplant, sliced

- 1 cup cherry tomatoes, diced
- 1/4 cup red onion, finely chopped
- 2 tablespoons fresh basil, chopped
- 1 tablespoon balsamic vinegar
- 1 tablespoon olive oil
- Salt and pepper to taste

Prep Time: 15 minutes

Cooking Time: 10 minutes

Serving Size: 1/2 cup

Serving Time: Dinner

Nutritional Information (per serving):

- Calories: 80
- Protein: 2g
- Fiber: 5g
- Healthy Fats: 5g

Directions:

1. Preheat the grill or grill pan.

2. Brush eggplant slices with olive oil, salt, and pepper. Grill for 4-5 minutes per side.
3. In a bowl, combine diced cherry tomatoes, red onion, basil, balsamic vinegar, olive oil, salt, and pepper.
4. Spoon tomato salsa over grilled eggplant before serving.

Serving Methods:

- Top with crumbled feta cheese.
- Serve as a side with grilled chicken or fish.

Quinoa and Black Bean Stuffed Peppers

A nutrient-dense side dish featuring colorful bell peppers stuffed with a mixture of quinoa, black beans, and spices, providing a satisfying and protein-packed addition to any meal.

Ingredients:

- 4 bell peppers, halved and seeds removed
- 1 cup cooked quinoa
- 1 cup black beans, drained and rinsed
- 1/2 cup corn kernels
- 1/4 cup red onion, finely chopped
- 1 teaspoon cumin
- 1/2 teaspoon chili powder
- Salt and pepper to taste

Prep Time: 20 minutes

Cooking Time: 25 minutes (includes baking time)

Serving Size: 1 half pepper

Serving Time: Dinner

Nutritional Information (per serving):

- Calories: 180
- Protein: 8g
- Fiber: 7g

- Healthy Fats: 3g

Directions:

1. Preheat the oven to 375°F (190°C).
2. In a bowl, mix cooked quinoa, black beans, corn, red onion, cumin, chili powder, salt, and pepper.
3. Stuff bell pepper halves with the quinoa and black bean mixture.
4. Bake for 25 minutes or until peppers are tender.
5. Serve with a side of salsa or guacamole.

Serving Methods:

- Top with a dollop of Greek yogurt.
- Serve with a side of mixed greens.

Garlic Roasted Broccoli

A simple and flavorful side dish featuring broccoli roasted with garlic and olive oil, creating a delicious and nutrient-rich addition to any meal.

Ingredients:

- 1 lb broccoli florets
- 3 cloves garlic, minced
- 2 tablespoons olive oil
- Salt and pepper to taste

Prep Time: 10 minutes

Cooking Time: 20 minutes

Serving Size: 1/2 cup

Serving Time: Dinner

Nutritional Information (per serving):

- Calories: 60
- Protein: 3g
- Fiber: 4g
- Healthy Fats: 4g

Directions:

1. Preheat the oven to 400°F (200°C).
2. Toss broccoli florets with minced garlic, olive oil, salt, and pepper.
3. Roast for 20 minutes or until broccoli is golden and slightly crispy.

Serving Methods:

- Squeeze fresh lemon juice before serving.
- Top with a sprinkle of grated Parmesan cheese.

Cauliflower and Chickpea Tabbouleh

A low-carb twist on the classic tabbouleh, featuring cauliflower and chickpeas tossed with fresh herbs and a lemony dressing, providing a light and refreshing side.

Ingredients:

- 1/2 head cauliflower, grated
- 1 can (15 oz) chickpeas, drained and rinsed
- 1 cup cucumber, diced
- 1 cup cherry tomatoes, halved
- 1/4 cup red onion, finely chopped
- 1/4 cup fresh parsley, chopped
- Juice of 2 lemons
- 2 tablespoons olive oil
- Salt and pepper to taste

Prep Time: 15 minutes

Cooking Time: 0 minutes

Serving Size: 1/2 cup

Serving Time: Lunch or Dinner

Nutritional Information (per serving):

- Calories: 120

- Protein: 4g
- Fiber: 5g
- Healthy Fats: 5g

Directions:

1. In a large bowl, combine grated cauliflower, chickpeas, cucumber, cherry tomatoes, red onion, and fresh parsley.
2. In a small bowl, whisk together lemon juice, olive oil, salt, and pepper.
3. Toss the tabbouleh with the lemony dressing just before serving.

Serving Methods:

- Serve as a side with grilled chicken or fish.
- Spoon over a bed of mixed greens for a salad variation.

Zucchini Noodles with Pesto

A light and low-carb side dish featuring zucchini noodles tossed in a vibrant basil pesto, creating a flavorful and nutrient-packed addition to any meal.

Ingredients:

- 4 medium zucchinis, spiralized
- 1 cup cherry tomatoes, halved
- 1/4 cup pine nuts, toasted
- 1/2 cup fresh basil leaves
- 1/4 cup Parmesan cheese, grated
- 2 cloves garlic
- 1/4 cup olive oil
- Salt and pepper to taste

Prep Time: 15 minutes

Cooking Time: 0 minutes

Serving Size: 1 cup

Serving Time: Lunch or Dinner

Nutritional Information (per serving):

- Calories: 150
- Protein: 4g
- Fiber: 3g
- Healthy Fats: 12g

Directions:

1. Spiralize zucchinis to create noodles.
2. In a blender, combine fresh basil, pine nuts, Parmesan cheese, garlic, and olive oil. Blend until smooth.
3. Toss zucchini noodles with pesto, cherry tomatoes, salt, and pepper.

Serving Methods:

- Top with grilled shrimp or chicken.
- Serve as a refreshing side alongside grilled fish.

Roasted Butternut Squash with Sage

A sweet and savory side dish featuring roasted butternut squash tossed with aromatic sage, providing a comforting and flavorful addition to fall and winter meals.

Ingredients:

- 1 medium butternut squash, peeled and diced
- 2 tablespoons olive oil
- 2 tablespoons fresh sage, chopped
- 1 tablespoon maple syrup
- Salt and pepper to taste

Prep Time: 15 minutes

Cooking Time: 30 minutes

Serving Size: 1/2 cup

Serving Time: Dinner

Nutritional Information (per serving):

- Calories: 90
- Protein: 1g
- Fiber: 4g
- Healthy Fats: 4g

Directions:

1. Preheat the oven to 400°F (200°C).
2. Toss diced butternut squash with olive oil, chopped sage, maple syrup, salt, and pepper.
3. Roast for 30 minutes or until squash is tender and caramelized.

Serving Methods:

- Sprinkle with crumbled goat cheese.
- Serve alongside grilled pork or chicken.

Asparagus and Tomato Frittata

A protein-packed side dish featuring a frittata with asparagus, cherry tomatoes, and eggs, creating a versatile and satisfying addition to breakfast or dinner.

Ingredients: 1 bunch asparagus, trimmed and cut into pieces

- 1 cup cherry tomatoes, halved
- 6 eggs, beaten
- 1/4 cup feta cheese, crumbled
- 1 tablespoon olive oil
- Salt and pepper to taste

Prep Time: 15 minutes

Cooking Time: 20 minutes

Serving Size: 1 wedge

Serving Time: Breakfast or Dinner

Nutritional Information (per serving):

- Calories: 120
- Protein: 9g
- Fiber: 2g
- Healthy Fats: 8g

Directions:

1. Preheat the oven to 375°F (190°C).
2. In an oven-safe skillet, sauté asparagus in olive oil until slightly tender.
3. Add cherry tomatoes and pour beaten eggs over the vegetables.
4. Sprinkle with crumbled feta cheese, salt, and pepper.
5. Bake for 20 minutes or until the frittata is set and slightly golden.

Serving Methods:

- Cut into wedges and serve with a side salad.
- Pair with whole-grain toast for a hearty breakfast.

Green Bean Almondine

A classic and elegant side dish featuring crisp green beans sautéed with garlic and toasted almonds, providing a flavorful and nutritious addition to any dinner.

Ingredients: 1 lb green beans, trimmed

- 2 tablespoons sliced almonds, toasted
- 2 cloves garlic, minced
- 1 tablespoon olive oil
- Juice of 1 lemon
- Salt and pepper to taste

Prep Time: 15 minutes

Cooking Time: 10 minutes

Serving Size: 1/2 cup

Serving Time: Dinner

Nutritional Information (per serving):

- Calories: 80
- Protein: 2g
- Fiber: 4g
- Healthy Fats: 5g

Directions:

1. Blanch green beans in boiling water for 2-3 minutes, then transfer to an ice bath.
2. In a skillet, sauté minced garlic in olive oil until fragrant.
3. Add blanched green beans and cook until tender-crisp.
4. Sprinkle with toasted almonds, squeeze lemon juice, and season with salt and pepper.

Serving Methods:

- Serve alongside grilled chicken or fish.
- Garnish with fresh chopped parsley.

Beet and Orange Salad

A vibrant and antioxidant-rich side dish featuring roasted beets and fresh oranges, tossed in a light vinaigrette, creating a colorful and refreshing addition to any meal.

Ingredients: 2 medium beets, roasted and diced

- 2 oranges, peeled and segmented
- 1/4 cup red onion, finely chopped
- 2 tablespoons balsamic vinegar
- 1 tablespoon olive oil
- 1 teaspoon honey
- Salt and pepper to taste

Prep Time: 20 minutes

Cooking Time: 40 minutes (for roasting beets)

Serving Size: 1/2 cup

Serving Time: Lunch or Dinner

Nutritional Information (per serving):

- Calories: 100
- Protein: 2g
- Fiber: 5g
- Healthy Fats: 4g

Directions:

1. Roast beets in the oven until tender, then dice.
2. In a bowl, combine diced beets, orange segments, and chopped red onion.
3. In a small bowl, whisk together balsamic vinegar, olive oil, honey, salt, and pepper.
4. Toss the salad with the vinaigrette just before serving.

Serving Methods:

- Crumble feta cheese on top.

- Serve over a bed of arugula or mixed greens.

Lemon Herb Roasted Potatoes

A comforting and flavorful side dish featuring baby potatoes roasted with a zesty lemon and herb seasoning, providing a delightful addition to any dinner.

Ingredients:

- 1 lb baby potatoes, halved
- 2 tablespoons olive oil
- Zest of 1 lemon
- 1 tablespoon fresh rosemary, chopped
- 1 tablespoon fresh thyme, chopped
- Salt and pepper to taste

Prep Time: 15 minutes

Cooking Time: 30 minutes

Serving Size: 1/2 cup

Serving Time: Dinner

Nutritional Information (per serving):

- Calories: 120
- Protein: 2g
- Fiber: 2g
- Healthy Fats: 5g

Directions:

1. Preheat the oven to 400°F (200°C).
2. Toss halved baby potatoes with olive oil, lemon zest, chopped rosemary, chopped thyme, salt, and pepper.
3. Roast for 30 minutes or until potatoes are golden and crispy.

Serving Methods:

- Sprinkle with chopped parsley.
- Serve alongside grilled steak or chicken.

Miso Glazed Eggplant

A savory and umami-packed side dish featuring eggplant glazed with a miso-based sauce, creating a flavorful and satisfying addition to any Asian-inspired meal.

Ingredients:

- 2 medium eggplants, sliced
- 2 tablespoons miso paste
- 1 tablespoon soy sauce
- 1 tablespoon rice vinegar
- 1 tablespoon sesame oil
- 1 tablespoon sesame seeds, toasted
- Green onions for garnish

Prep Time: 15 minutes

Cooking Time: 20 minutes

Serving Size: 1/2 cup

Serving Time: Dinner

Nutritional Information (per serving):

- Calories: 100
- Protein: 2g
- Fiber: 6g
- Healthy Fats: 5g

Directions:

1. Preheat the oven to 400°F (200°C).
2. In a bowl, whisk together miso paste, soy sauce, rice vinegar, and sesame oil.
3. Brush eggplant slices with the miso glaze and roast for 20 minutes or until tender.
4. Sprinkle with toasted sesame seeds and garnish with sliced green onions.

Serving Methods:

- Serve over a bed of brown rice.
- Pair with grilled tofu or salmon.

SALAD RECIPES

Mediterranean Quinoa Salad

A refreshing and protein-packed salad featuring quinoa, cherry tomatoes, cucumber, olives, and feta cheese, tossed in a zesty Mediterranean dressing.

Ingredients:

- 1 cup quinoa, cooked
- 1 cup cherry tomatoes, halved
- 1 cucumber, diced
- 1/4 cup Kalamata olives, sliced
- 1/4 cup feta cheese, crumbled
- 2 tablespoons olive oil
- Juice of 1 lemon
- Fresh oregano for garnish
- Salt and pepper to taste

Prep Time: 15 minutes

Cooking Time: 15 minutes (for quinoa)

Serving Size: 1 cup

Serving Time: Lunch or Dinner

Nutritional Information (per serving):

- Calories: 180
- Protein: 6g
- Fiber: 4g
- Healthy Fats: 8g

Directions:

1. In a large bowl, combine cooked quinoa, cherry tomatoes, cucumber, Kalamata olives, and feta cheese.
2. In a small bowl, whisk together olive oil, lemon juice, salt, and pepper.

3. Toss the salad with the dressing and garnish with fresh oregano.

Serving Methods:

- Top with grilled chicken or shrimp.
- Serve alongside a piece of whole-grain bread.

Spinach and Berry Salad

A vibrant and antioxidant-rich salad featuring fresh spinach, mixed berries, goat cheese, and walnuts, drizzled with a light balsamic vinaigrette.

Ingredients:

- 4 cups fresh spinach leaves
- 1 cup mixed berries (strawberries, blueberries, raspberries)
- 1/4 cup goat cheese, crumbled
- 1/4 cup walnuts, chopped
- 2 tablespoons balsamic vinegar
- 1 tablespoon olive oil
- 1 teaspoon honey
- Salt and pepper to taste

Prep Time: 10 minutes

Cooking Time: 0 minutes

Serving Size: 1 cup

Serving Time: Lunch or Dinner

Nutritional Information (per serving):

- Calories: 120
- Protein: 4g
- Fiber: 3g
- Healthy Fats: 8g

Directions:

1. In a large bowl, combine fresh spinach, mixed berries, goat cheese, and chopped walnuts.

2. In a small bowl, whisk together balsamic vinegar, olive oil, honey, salt, and pepper.
3. Drizzle the vinaigrette over the salad just before serving.

Serving Methods:

- Add grilled chicken or salmon on top.
- Serve as a side with a quinoa bowl.

Shrimp and Avocado Salad

A protein-rich salad featuring succulent shrimp, creamy avocado, cherry tomatoes, and arugula, dressed in a citrusy lime vinaigrette.

Ingredients:

- 8 oz shrimp, peeled and deveined
- 1 avocado, diced
- 1 cup cherry tomatoes, halved
- 2 cups arugula
- 1 lime, juiced
- 2 tablespoons olive oil
- 1 teaspoon Dijon mustard
- Salt and pepper to taste

Prep Time: 15 minutes

Cooking Time: 5 minutes

Serving Size: 1 cup

Serving Time: Lunch or Dinner

Nutritional Information (per serving):

- Calories: 250
- Protein: 15g
- Fiber: 5g
- Healthy Fats: 18g

Directions:

1. Season shrimp with salt and pepper, then sauté in olive oil until cooked.
2. In a large bowl, combine cooked shrimp, diced avocado, cherry tomatoes, and arugula.
3. In a small bowl, whisk together lime juice, olive oil, Dijon mustard, salt, and pepper.
4. Toss the salad with the lime vinaigrette just before serving.

Serving Methods:

- Serve over a bed of quinoa or brown rice.
- Top with a sprinkle of feta cheese.

Grilled Chicken Caesar Salad

A classic Caesar salad with a twist, featuring grilled chicken, crisp romaine lettuce, cherry tomatoes, and homemade whole-grain croutons.

Ingredients:

- 2 boneless, skinless chicken breasts
- 1 head romaine lettuce, chopped
- 1 cup cherry tomatoes, halved
- 1/4 cup Parmesan cheese, grated
- Whole-grain croutons
- 1/4 cup plain Greek yogurt
- 2 tablespoons olive oil
- 1 tablespoon Dijon mustard
- 1 clove garlic, minced
- Juice of 1 lemon
- Salt and pepper to taste

Prep Time: 15 minutes

Cooking Time: 15 minutes

Serving Size: 1.5 cups

Serving Time: Lunch or Dinner

Nutritional Information (per serving):

- Calories: 320
- Protein: 30g
- Fiber: 6g
- Healthy Fats: 15g

Directions:

1. Season chicken breasts with salt and pepper, then grill until fully cooked.
2. In a large bowl, combine chopped romaine lettuce, cherry tomatoes, Parmesan cheese, and whole-grain croutons.
3. Slice grilled chicken and add to the salad.
4. In a small bowl, whisk together Greek yogurt, olive oil, Dijon mustard, minced garlic, lemon juice, salt, and pepper.
5. Drizzle the Caesar dressing over the salad and toss before serving.

Serving Methods:

- Sprinkle with additional Parmesan cheese.
- Serve with a side of multigrain bread.

Caprese Salad with Balsamic Glaze

A classic Caprese salad featuring ripe tomatoes, fresh mozzarella, and basil, drizzled with a balsamic glaze for a simple yet flavorful dish.

Ingredients: 4 large tomatoes, sliced

- 1 ball fresh mozzarella, sliced
- Fresh basil leaves
- Balsamic glaze
- Olive oil
- Salt and pepper to taste

Prep Time: 10 minutes

Cooking Time: 0 minutes

Serving Size: 1 cup

Serving Time: Lunch or Dinner

Nutritional Information (per serving):

- Calories: 180
- Protein: 10g
- Fiber: 3g
- Healthy Fats: 12g

Directions:

1. Arrange tomato and mozzarella slices on a serving platter.
2. Tuck fresh basil leaves between tomato and mozzarella slices.
3. Drizzle with balsamic glaze and olive oil.
4. Sprinkle with salt and pepper to taste.

Serving Methods:

- Serve as a side with grilled chicken or fish.
- Top with a handful of pine nuts for added crunch.

Asian-Inspired Chicken Salad

A vibrant and flavorful salad featuring shredded chicken, cabbage, carrots, edamame, and a sesame-ginger dressing for an Asian-inspired twist.

Ingredients: 2 cups shredded cooked chicken

- 2 cups shredded cabbage, 1 cup shredded carrots
- 1 cup edamame, cooked
- 1/4 cup green onions, sliced
- 2 tablespoons sesame seeds
- Sesame-ginger dressing

Prep Time: 15 minutes

Cooking Time: 0 minutes

Serving Size: 1.5 cups

Serving Time: Lunch or Dinner

Nutritional Information (per serving):

- Calories: 280, Protein: 24g
- Fiber: 8g, Healthy Fats: 12g

Directions:

1. In a large bowl, combine shredded chicken, shredded cabbage, shredded carrots, edamame, green onions, and sesame seeds.
2. Toss the salad with sesame-ginger dressing just before serving.

Serving Methods:

- Top with crispy wonton strips.
- Serve with a side of brown rice.

Tuna and White Bean Salad

A protein-packed salad featuring flaked tuna, white beans, cherry tomatoes, and arugula, tossed in a lemon-herb vinaigrette.

Ingredients: 2 cans (5 oz each) tuna, drained

- 1 can (15 oz) white beans, drained and rinsed
- 1 cup cherry tomatoes, halved
- 2 cups arugula
- 2 tablespoons fresh parsley, chopped
- 2 tablespoons olive oil
- Juice of 1 lemon
- Salt and pepper to taste

Prep Time: 10 minutes

Cooking Time: 0 minutes

Serving Size: 1.5 cups

Serving Time: Lunch or Dinner

Nutritional Information (per serving):

- Calories: 250
- Protein: 25g

- Fiber: 8g
- Healthy Fats: 10g

Directions:

1. In a large bowl, combine flaked tuna, white beans, cherry tomatoes, arugula, and fresh parsley.
2. In a small bowl, whisk together olive oil, lemon juice, salt, and pepper.
3. Toss the salad with the lemon-herb vinaigrette just before serving.

Serving Methods:

- Serve over a bed of mixed greens.
- Spoon onto whole-grain crackers for a light snack.

Roasted Vegetable Quinoa Salad

A hearty and nutrient-rich salad featuring roasted vegetables, quinoa, chickpeas, and a lemon-tahini dressing for a satisfying and flavorful meal.

Ingredients: 1 cup quinoa, cooked

- 2 cups mixed roasted vegetables (zucchini, bell peppers, cherry tomatoes)
- 1 can (15 oz) chickpeas, drained and rinsed
- 1/4 cup red onion, finely chopped
- 2 tablespoons fresh parsley, chopped
- Lemon-tahini dressing

Prep Time: 20 minutes

Cooking Time: 20 minutes (for quinoa and roasting vegetables)

Serving Size: 1.5 cups

Serving Time: Lunch or Dinner

Nutritional Information (per serving):

- Calories: 320
- Protein: 12g

- Fiber: 8g
- Healthy Fats: 10g

Directions:

1. In a large bowl, combine cooked quinoa, roasted vegetables, chickpeas, red onion, and fresh parsley.
2. Toss the salad with lemon-tahini dressing just before serving.

Serving Methods:

- Top with grilled chicken or tofu.
- Serve chilled as a refreshing summer meal.

Waldorf Chicken Salad

A classic Waldorf salad with a protein boost, featuring diced chicken, crisp apples, celery, grapes, and walnuts, dressed in a yogurt-mayonnaise dressing.

Ingredients:

- 2 cups diced cooked chicken
- 2 apples, diced
- 1 cup celery, chopped
- 1 cup red grapes, halved
- 1/2 cup walnuts, chopped
- 1/2 cup plain Greek yogurt
- 2 tablespoons mayonnaise
- 1 tablespoon honey
- Salt and pepper to taste

Prep Time: 15 minutes

Cooking Time: 0 minutes

Serving Size: 1.5 cups

Serving Time: Lunch or Dinner

Nutritional Information (per serving):

- Calories: 290

- Protein: 20g
- Fiber: 5g
- Healthy Fats: 15g

Directions:

1. In a large bowl, combine diced chicken, diced apples, chopped celery, halved grapes, and chopped walnuts.
2. In a small bowl, whisk together Greek yogurt, mayonnaise, honey, salt, and pepper.
3. Toss the salad with the yogurt-mayonnaise dressing just before serving.

Serving Methods:

- Serve over a bed of mixed greens.
- Spoon onto whole-grain wraps for a light lunch.

Roasted Beet and Goat Cheese Salad

A colorful and flavorful salad featuring roasted beets, creamy goat cheese, mixed greens, and a balsamic vinaigrette for a delightful and sophisticated dish.

Ingredients:

- 2 medium beets, roasted and sliced
- 2 cups mixed salad greens
- 1/4 cup goat cheese, crumbled
- 2 tablespoons balsamic vinegar
- 1 tablespoon olive oil
- 1 teaspoon Dijon mustard
- Salt and pepper to taste

Prep Time: 20 minutes

Cooking Time: 40 minutes (for roasting beets)

Serving Size: 1.5 cups

Serving Time: Lunch or Dinner

Nutritional Information (per serving):

- Calories: 200
- Protein: 8g
- Fiber: 5g
- Healthy Fats: 10g

Directions:

1. Roast beets in the oven until tender, then slice.
2. In a large bowl, combine roasted beet slices, mixed salad greens, and crumbled goat cheese.
3. In a small bowl, whisk together balsamic vinegar, olive oil, Dijon mustard, salt, and pepper.
4. Toss the salad with the balsamic vinaigrette just before serving.

Serving Methods:

- Top with grilled chicken or salmon.
- Serve with a side of whole-grain bread.

Superfood Kale Salad with Citrus Vinaigrette

A nutrient-packed salad featuring kale, quinoa, blueberries, walnuts, and a zesty citrus vinaigrette for a refreshing and hearty dish.

Ingredients:

- 4 cups kale, chopped
- 1 cup cooked quinoa
- 1/2 cup blueberries
- 1/4 cup walnuts, chopped
- 1/4 cup feta cheese, crumbled
- Citrus Vinaigrette (olive oil, orange juice, lemon juice, Dijon mustard, honey)
- Salt and pepper to taste

Prep Time: 15 minutes

Cooking Time: 15 minutes (for quinoa)

Serving Size: 1.5 cups

Serving Time: Lunch or Dinner

Nutritional Information (per serving):

- Calories: 280
- Protein: 9g
- Fiber: 6g
- Healthy Fats: 14g

Directions:

1. Massage kale with a bit of olive oil to soften.
2. In a large bowl, combine kale, cooked quinoa, blueberries, chopped walnuts, and crumbled feta.
3. Whisk together the ingredients for the citrus vinaigrette and drizzle over the salad.
4. Toss well and season with salt and pepper.

Serving Methods:

- Top with grilled chicken or tofu.
- Serve with a side of whole-grain crackers.

Salmon and Avocado Caesar Salad

A protein-rich twist on the classic Caesar salad, featuring grilled salmon, creamy avocado, romaine lettuce, and a light Greek yogurt Caesar dressing.

Ingredients:

- 8 oz salmon fillet, grilled and flaked
- 1 avocado, sliced
- 1 head romaine lettuce, chopped
- Whole-grain croutons
- Greek Yogurt Caesar Dressing (Greek yogurt, Parmesan cheese, anchovy paste, garlic, lemon juice)
- Salt and pepper to taste

Prep Time: 15 minutes

Cooking Time: 10 minutes

Serving Size: 1.5 cups

Serving Time: Lunch or Dinner

Nutritional Information (per serving):

- Calories: 320
- Protein: 25g
- Fiber: 6g
- Healthy Fats: 15g

Directions:

1. In a large bowl, combine grilled and flaked salmon, sliced avocado, chopped romaine lettuce, and whole-grain croutons.
2. Whisk together the ingredients for the Greek yogurt Caesar dressing and drizzle over the salad.
3. Toss well and season with salt and pepper.

Serving Methods:

- Sprinkle with additional Parmesan cheese.
- Serve with a side of multigrain bread.

Beet and Quinoa Power Salad

A vibrant and protein-packed salad featuring roasted beets, quinoa, arugula, goat cheese, and a balsamic vinaigrette for a delicious and energizing meal.

Ingredients:

- 2 medium beets, roasted and diced
- 1 cup cooked quinoa
- 2 cups arugula
- 1/4 cup goat cheese, crumbled
- 2 tablespoons balsamic vinegar
- 1 tablespoon olive oil

- 1 teaspoon honey
- Salt and pepper to taste

Prep Time: 20 minutes

Cooking Time: 40 minutes (for roasting beets)

Serving Size: 1.5 cups

Serving Time: Lunch or Dinner

Nutritional Information (per serving):

- Calories: 240
- Protein: 8g
- Fiber: 6g
- Healthy Fats: 10g

Directions:

1. Roast beets in the oven until tender, then dice.
2. In a large bowl, combine roasted beet cubes, cooked quinoa, arugula, and crumbled goat cheese.
3. In a small bowl, whisk together balsamic vinegar, olive oil, honey, salt, and pepper.
4. Toss the salad with the balsamic vinaigrette just before serving.

Serving Methods:

- Top with grilled chicken or tofu.
- Serve with a side of whole-grain bread.

Chickpea and Tomato Summer Salad

A light and refreshing salad featuring chickpeas, cherry tomatoes, cucumber, and fresh herbs, tossed in a lemon-tahini dressing for a perfect summer dish.

Ingredients:

- 1 can (15 oz) chickpeas, drained and rinsed
- 1 cup cherry tomatoes, halved
- 1 cucumber, diced

- 1/4 cup red onion, finely chopped
- 2 tablespoons fresh parsley, chopped
- Lemon-Tahini Dressing (tahini, lemon juice, olive oil, garlic, honey)
- Salt and pepper to taste

Prep Time: 15 minutes

Cooking Time: 0 minutes

Serving Size: 1.5 cups

Serving Time: Lunch or Dinner

Nutritional Information (per serving):

- Calories: 220
- Protein: 8g
- Fiber: 8g
- Healthy Fats: 10g

Directions:

1. In a large bowl, combine chickpeas, cherry tomatoes, diced cucumber, chopped red onion, and fresh parsley.
2. Whisk together the ingredients for the lemon-tahini dressing and drizzle over the salad.
3. Toss well and season with salt and pepper.

Serving Methods:

- Top with grilled shrimp or salmon.
- Serve over a bed of mixed greens.

Quinoa and Mango Summer Salad

A tropical-inspired salad featuring quinoa, ripe mango, avocado, and a cilantro-lime dressing for a burst of flavors and textures.

Ingredients: 1 cup cooked quinoa

- 1 ripe mango, diced
- 1 avocado, sliced

- 1/4 cup red bell pepper, diced
- 2 tablespoons fresh cilantro, chopped
- Cilantro-Lime Dressing (lime juice, olive oil, honey, garlic)
- Salt and pepper to taste

Prep Time: 20 minutes

Cooking Time: 15 minutes

Serving Size: 1.5 cups

Serving Time: Lunch or Dinner

Nutritional Information (per serving):

- Calories: 280
- Protein: 6g
- Fiber: 7g
- Healthy Fats: 15g

Directions:

1. In a large bowl, combine cooked quinoa, diced mango, sliced avocado, diced red bell pepper, and chopped cilantro.
2. Whisk together the ingredients for the cilantro-lime dressing and drizzle over the salad.
3. Toss well and season with salt and pepper.

Serving Methods:

- Top with grilled chicken or tofu.
- Serve as a side with fish tacos.

Pomegranate and Walnut Spinach Salad

A festive and antioxidant-rich salad featuring spinach, pomegranate seeds, walnuts, and goat cheese, drizzled with a balsamic vinaigrette for a delightful holiday meal.

Ingredients: 4 cups fresh spinach leaves

- 1/2 cup pomegranate seeds
- 1/4 cup walnuts, chopped

139

- 1/4 cup goat cheese, crumbled
- Balsamic Vinaigrette (balsamic vinegar, olive oil, Dijon mustard, honey)
- Salt and pepper to taste

Prep Time: 15 minutes

Cooking Time: 0 minutes

Serving Size: 1.5 cups

Serving Time: Lunch or Dinner

Nutritional Information (per serving):

- Calories: 260
- Protein: 8g
- Fiber: 5g
- Healthy Fats: 15g

Directions:

1. In a large bowl, combine fresh spinach leaves, pomegranate seeds, chopped walnuts, and crumbled goat cheese.
2. Whisk together the ingredients for the balsamic vinaigrette and drizzle over the salad.
3. Toss well and season with salt and pepper.

Serving Methods:

- Top with grilled chicken or salmon.
- Serve as a side with a holiday roast.

Southwest Black Bean and Corn Salad

A colorful and protein-rich salad featuring black beans, corn, tomatoes, and avocado, tossed in a cilantro-lime dressing for a Southwestern flair.

Ingredients: 1 can (15 oz) black beans, drained and rinsed

- 1 cup corn kernels (fresh or thawed)
- 1 cup cherry tomatoes, halved
- 1 avocado, diced

- 1/4 cup red onion, finely chopped
- 2 tablespoons fresh cilantro, chopped
- Cilantro-Lime Dressing (lime juice, olive oil, garlic, cumin)
- Salt and pepper to taste

Prep Time: 15 minutes

Cooking Time: 0 minutes

Serving Size: 1.5 cups

Serving Time: Lunch or Dinner

Nutritional Information (per serving):

- Calories: 290
- Protein: 10g
- Fiber: 10g
- Healthy Fats: 15g

Directions:

1. In a large bowl, combine black beans, corn kernels, cherry tomatoes, diced avocado, chopped red onion, and chopped cilantro.
2. Whisk together the ingredients for the cilantro-lime dressing and drizzle over the salad.
3. Toss well and season with salt and pepper.

Serving Methods:

- Top with grilled shrimp or chicken.
- Serve as a side with tortilla chips.

Greek Orzo Salad with Feta

A Mediterranean-inspired salad featuring orzo pasta, cherry tomatoes, cucumber, olives, and feta cheese, dressed in a lemon-oregano vinaigrette.

Ingredients: 1 cup orzo pasta, cooked

- 1 cup cherry tomatoes, halved

- 1 cucumber, diced
- 1/4 cup Kalamata olives, sliced
- 1/4 cup feta cheese, crumbled
- Lemon-Oregano Vinaigrette (lemon juice, olive oil, oregano, garlic)
- Salt and pepper to taste

Prep Time: 20 minutes

Cooking Time: 10 minutes (for orzo)

Serving Size: 1.5 cups

Serving Time: Lunch or Dinner

Nutritional Information (per serving):

- Calories: 280, Protein: 8g
- Fiber: 4g, Healthy Fats: 12g

Directions:

1. Cook orzo according to package instructions and let it cool.
2. In a large bowl, combine cooked orzo, cherry tomatoes, diced cucumber, sliced Kalamata olives, and crumbled feta cheese.
3. Whisk together the ingredients for the lemon-oregano vinaigrette and drizzle over the salad.
4. Toss well and season with salt and pepper.

Serving Methods:

- Top with grilled chicken or lamb.
- Serve as a refreshing side with grilled fish.

Apple and Walnut Chicken Salad

A satisfying and protein-packed salad featuring grilled chicken, crisp apples, walnuts, and a honey-mustard dressing for a delightful combination of flavors.

Ingredients: 2 boneless, skinless chicken breasts, grilled and sliced

- 2 apples, thinly sliced

- 1/4 cup walnuts, chopped
- 2 cups mixed salad greens
- Honey-Mustard Dressing (dijon mustard, honey, olive oil)
- Salt and pepper to taste

Prep Time: 15 minutes

Cooking Time: 15 minutes

Serving Size: 1.5 cups

Serving Time: Lunch or Dinner

Nutritional Information (per serving):

- Calories: 310
- Protein: 24g
- Fiber: 6g
- Healthy Fats: 16g

Directions:

1. Grill chicken breasts until fully cooked, then slice.
2. In a large bowl, combine grilled chicken slices, thinly sliced apples, chopped walnuts, and mixed salad greens.
3. Whisk together the ingredients for the honey-mustard dressing and drizzle over the salad.
4. Toss well and season with salt and pepper.

Serving Methods:

- Top with crumbled blue cheese.
- Serve with a side of whole-grain bread.

Quinoa and Broccoli Detox Salad

A cleansing and nutrient-rich salad featuring quinoa, broccoli, almonds, and a lemon-turmeric dressing for a detoxifying and delicious meal.

Ingredients: 1 cup cooked quinoa

- 2 cups broccoli florets, blanched
- 1/4 cup almonds, sliced

- 1/4 cup dried cranberries
- Lemon-Turmeric Dressing (lemon juice, olive oil, turmeric, ginger)
- Salt and pepper to taste

Prep Time: 20 minutes

Cooking Time: 15 minutes

Serving Size: 1.5 cups

Serving Time: Lunch or Dinner

Nutritional Information (per serving):

- Calories: 270
- Protein: 8g
- Fiber: 7g
- Healthy Fats: 14g

Directions:

1. Cook quinoa according to package instructions and let it cool.
2. Blanch broccoli florets in boiling water for 2 minutes, then plunge into ice water.
3. In a large bowl, combine cooked quinoa, blanched broccoli, sliced almonds, and dried cranberries.
4. Whisk together the ingredients for the lemon-turmeric dressing and drizzle over the salad.
5. Toss well and season with salt and pepper.

Serving Methods:

- Top with grilled tofu or shrimp.
- Serve as a light and detoxifying lunch.

SOUP RECIPES

Quinoa and Vegetable Minestrone Soup

A hearty and nutrient-packed minestrone soup featuring quinoa, a variety of vegetables, and aromatic Italian herbs for a comforting and balanced meal.

Ingredients:

- 1 cup quinoa, uncooked
- 4 cups mixed vegetables (carrots, celery, zucchini, tomatoes), diced
- 1 can (15 oz) kidney beans, drained and rinsed
- 1 onion, chopped
- 4 cloves garlic, minced
- 8 cups vegetable broth
- 2 teaspoons Italian seasoning
- Salt and pepper to taste

Prep Time: 15 minutes

Cooking Time: 30 minutes

Serving Size: 1 cup

Serving Time: Lunch or Dinner

Nutritional Information (per serving):

- Calories: 180
- Protein: 8g
- Fiber: 6g
- Healthy Fats: 2g

Directions:

1. Rinse quinoa under cold water.
2. In a large pot, sauté onion and garlic until softened.
3. Add diced vegetables, kidney beans, quinoa, vegetable broth, Italian seasoning, salt, and pepper.

145

4. Bring to a boil, then simmer for 25-30 minutes until vegetables are tender.
5. Adjust seasoning and serve hot.

Serving Methods:

- Garnish with freshly chopped parsley.
- Serve with a side of whole-grain bread.

Lentil and Spinach Soup

A protein-rich and iron-packed soup featuring lentils, spinach, and tomatoes, seasoned with cumin and coriander for a flavorful and nutritious option.

Ingredients:

- 1 cup dried green or brown lentils, rinsed
- 4 cups fresh spinach leaves
- 1 can (15 oz) diced tomatoes
- 1 onion, chopped
- 3 cloves garlic, minced
- 8 cups vegetable broth
- 1 teaspoon ground cumin
- 1 teaspoon ground coriander
- Salt and pepper to taste

Prep Time: 10 minutes

Cooking Time: 40 minutes

Serving Size: 1 cup

Serving Time: Lunch or Dinner

Nutritional Information (per serving):

- Calories: 200
- Protein: 14g
- Fiber: 8g
- Healthy Fats: 1g

Directions:

1. In a large pot, sauté onion and garlic until translucent.
2. Add lentils, diced tomatoes, vegetable broth, cumin, coriander, salt, and pepper.
3. Bring to a boil, then reduce heat and simmer for 35-40 minutes.
4. Stir in fresh spinach and cook until wilted.
5. Adjust seasoning and serve hot.

Serving Methods:

- Squeeze a splash of fresh lemon juice before serving.
- Serve with a dollop of Greek yogurt.

Chicken and Wild Rice Soup

A comforting and protein-packed soup featuring tender chicken, wild rice, carrots, and celery, seasoned with thyme and rosemary for a homely flavor.

Ingredients:

- 1 cup wild rice, uncooked
- 2 cups cooked chicken breast, shredded
- 4 carrots, diced
- 3 celery stalks, chopped
- 1 onion, finely chopped
- 4 cloves garlic, minced
- 8 cups chicken broth
- 1 teaspoon dried thyme
- 1 teaspoon dried rosemary
- Salt and pepper to taste

Prep Time: 20 minutes

Cooking Time: 45 minutes

Serving Size: 1 cup

Serving Time: Lunch or Dinner

Nutritional Information (per serving):

- Calories: 220
- Protein: 18g
- Fiber: 4g
- Healthy Fats: 3g

Directions:

1. Cook wild rice according to package instructions.
2. In a large pot, sauté onion and garlic until fragrant.
3. Add carrots, celery, shredded chicken, cooked wild rice, chicken broth, thyme, rosemary, salt, and pepper.
4. Simmer for 35-40 minutes until vegetables are tender.
5. Adjust seasoning and serve hot.

Serving Methods:

- Garnish with fresh parsley.
- Serve with a slice of whole-grain bread.

Tomato Basil Quinoa Soup

A flavorful and protein-packed tomato soup featuring quinoa, fresh basil, and a hint of Parmesan for a nutritious and satisfying option.

Ingredients:

- 1 cup quinoa, uncooked
- 1 can (28 oz) crushed tomatoes
- 1 onion, chopped
- 3 cloves garlic, minced
- 8 cups vegetable broth
- 1 cup fresh basil, chopped
- 1/4 cup grated Parmesan cheese
- Salt and pepper to taste

Prep Time: 15 minutes

Cooking Time: 30 minutes

Serving Size: 1 cup

Serving Time: Lunch or Dinner

Nutritional Information (per serving):

- Calories: 190
- Protein: 8g
- Fiber: 5g
- Healthy Fats: 2g

Directions:

1. Rinse quinoa under cold water.
2. In a large pot, sauté onion and garlic until softened.
3. Add crushed tomatoes, vegetable broth, quinoa, salt, and pepper.
4. Bring to a boil, then simmer for 25-30 minutes.
5. Stir in fresh basil and Parmesan cheese before serving.

Serving Methods:

- Drizzle with balsamic glaze.
- Serve with a side of whole-grain crackers.

Butternut Squash and Apple Soup

A sweet and savory soup featuring roasted butternut squash, apples, and warming spices like cinnamon and nutmeg for a comforting and immune-boosting dish.

Ingredients:

- 1 medium butternut squash, peeled and diced
- 2 apples, cored and chopped
- 1 onion, chopped
- 3 cloves garlic, minced
- 4 cups vegetable broth
- 1 teaspoon ground cinnamon
- 1/2 teaspoon ground nutmeg
- Salt and pepper to taste

Prep Time: 20 minutes

Cooking Time: 40 minutes

Serving Size: 1 cup

Serving Time: Lunch or Dinner

Nutritional Information (per serving):

- Calories: 150
- Protein: 2g
- Fiber: 5g
- Healthy Fats: 1g

Directions:

1. Preheat the oven to 400°F (200°C).
2. Place diced butternut squash and chopped apples on a baking sheet, drizzle with olive oil, and roast for 25-30 minutes.
3. In a large pot, sauté onion and garlic until translucent.
4. Add roasted butternut squash, apples, vegetable broth, cinnamon, nutmeg, salt, and pepper.
5. Simmer for 15-20 minutes, then blend until smooth.

Serving Methods:

- Garnish with a dollop of Greek yogurt.
- Serve with a sprinkle of toasted pumpkin seeds.

Spinach and White Bean Soup

A protein and fiber-rich soup featuring white beans, spinach, tomatoes, and Italian herbs for a light yet satisfying option.

Ingredients: 2 cans (15 oz each) cannellini beans, drained and rinsed

- 4 cups fresh spinach leaves
- 1 can (14 oz) diced tomatoes
- 1 onion, chopped
- 3 cloves garlic, minced
- 8 cups vegetable broth

- 1 teaspoon dried oregano
- 1 teaspoon dried thyme
- Salt and pepper to taste

Prep Time: 15 minutes

Cooking Time: 30 minutes

Serving Size: 1 cup

Serving Time: Lunch or Dinner

Nutritional Information (per serving):

- Calories: 170
- Protein: 9g
- Fiber: 6g
- Healthy Fats: 1g

Directions:

1. In a large pot, sauté onion and garlic until softened.
2. Add cannellini beans, diced tomatoes, vegetable broth, spinach, oregano, thyme, salt, and pepper.
3. Bring to a boil, then simmer for 25-30 minutes.
4. Adjust seasoning and serve hot.

Serving Methods:

1. Sprinkle with grated Parmesan cheese.
2. Serve with a slice of whole-grain baguette.

Miso and Mushroom Soup

An umami-packed and gut-friendly soup featuring miso paste, shiitake mushrooms, tofu, and green onions for a delicious and probiotic-rich option.

Ingredients: 1/4 cup miso paste

- 8 cups vegetable broth
- 1 cup shiitake mushrooms, sliced
- 1 block firm tofu, diced

- 3 green onions, chopped
- 2 tablespoons soy sauce
- 1 teaspoon sesame oil

Prep Time: 15 minutes

Cooking Time: 20 minutes

Serving Size: 1 cup

Serving Time: Lunch or Dinner

Nutritional Information (per serving):

- Calories: 120
- Protein: 8g
- Fiber: 2g
- Healthy Fats: 6g

Directions:

1. In a small bowl, dissolve miso paste in a bit of warm water.
2. In a pot, bring vegetable broth to a simmer and add miso paste, shiitake mushrooms, tofu, soy sauce, and sesame oil.
3. Simmer for 15-20 minutes, then garnish with chopped green onions.
4. Serve hot.

Serving Methods:

- Add a dash of sriracha for heat.
- Serve with a side of brown rice.

Turmeric and Ginger Carrot Soup

An anti-inflammatory and immune-boosting soup featuring carrots, turmeric, ginger, and coconut milk for a vibrant and nutritious option.

Ingredients: 6 cups carrots, chopped

- 1 onion, chopped
- 3 cloves garlic, minced
- 2 teaspoons ground turmeric

- 1 teaspoon fresh ginger, grated
- 1 can (14 oz) coconut milk
- 8 cups vegetable broth
- Salt and pepper to taste

Prep Time: 15 minutes

Cooking Time: 30 minutes

Serving Size: 1 cup

Serving Time: Lunch or Dinner

Nutritional Information (per serving):

- Calories: 160
- Protein: 2g
- Fiber: 5g
- Healthy Fats: 9g

Directions:

1. In a large pot, sauté onion and garlic until softened.
2. Add chopped carrots, ground turmeric, fresh ginger, vegetable broth, and coconut milk.
3. Bring to a boil, then simmer for 25-30 minutes.
4. Blend until smooth, season with salt and pepper, and serve hot.

Serving Methods:

- Drizzle with a swirl of coconut cream.
- Serve with a sprinkle of chopped cilantro.

Cabbage and White Bean Soup

A low-calorie and fiber-rich soup featuring cabbage, white beans, tomatoes, and herbs for a filling and weight-friendly option.

Ingredients: 1/2 head green cabbage, shredded

- 2 cans (15 oz each) cannellini beans, drained and rinsed
- 1 can (14 oz) diced tomatoes
- 1 onion, chopped

153

- 3 cloves garlic, minced
- 8 cups vegetable broth
- 1 teaspoon dried thyme
- 1 teaspoon smoked paprika
- Salt and pepper to taste

Prep Time: 15 minutes

Cooking Time: 30 minutes

Serving Size: 1 cup

Serving Time: Lunch or Dinner

Nutritional Information (per serving):

- Calories: 140
- Protein: 8g
- Fiber: 6g
- Healthy Fats: 1g

Directions:

1. In a large pot, sauté onion and garlic until softened.
2. Add shredded cabbage, cannellini beans, diced tomatoes, vegetable broth, thyme, smoked paprika, salt, and pepper.
3. Bring to a boil, then simmer for 25-30 minutes.
4. Adjust seasoning and serve hot.

Serving Methods:

- Sprinkle with nutritional yeast.
- Serve with a side of whole-grain crackers.

Chicken and Barley Vegetable Soup

A wholesome and protein-rich soup featuring barley, lean chicken, a medley of vegetables, and savory herbs for a comforting and balanced meal.

Ingredients: 1 cup barley, uncooked

- 2 cups cooked chicken breast, shredded

- 4 carrots, diced
- 3 celery stalks, chopped
- 1 onion, finely chopped
- 4 cloves garlic, minced
- 8 cups chicken broth
- 1 teaspoon dried thyme
- 1 teaspoon dried rosemary
- Salt and pepper to taste

Prep Time: 20 minutes

Cooking Time: 45 minutes

Serving Size: 1 cup

Serving Time: Lunch or Dinner

Nutritional Information (per serving):

- Calories: 210
- Protein: 16g
- Fiber: 6g
- Healthy Fats: 2g

Directions:

1. Cook barley according to package instructions.
2. In a large pot, sauté onion and garlic until fragrant.
3. Add diced carrots, celery, shredded chicken, cooked barley, chicken broth, thyme, rosemary, salt, and pepper.
4. Simmer for 35-40 minutes until vegetables are tender.
5. Adjust seasoning and serve hot.

Serving Methods:

- Garnish with chopped fresh parsley.
- Serve with a slice of whole-grain bread.

Sweet Potato and Kale Lentil Soup

A nutrient-dense soup featuring sweet potatoes, lentils, and kale, providing a rich source of vitamins, minerals, and fiber for overall health and metabolic support.

Ingredients:

- 1 cup dried green or brown lentils, rinsed
- 2 sweet potatoes, peeled and diced
- 4 cups kale, chopped
- 1 onion, finely chopped
- 3 cloves garlic, minced
- 8 cups vegetable broth
- 1 teaspoon cumin
- 1/2 teaspoon smoked paprika
- Salt and pepper to taste

Prep Time: 15 minutes

Cooking Time: 40 minutes

Serving Size: 1 cup

Serving Time: Lunch or Dinner

Nutritional Information (per serving):

- Calories: 220
- Protein: 12g
- Fiber: 10g
- Healthy Fats: 1g

Directions:

1. In a large pot, sauté onion and garlic until translucent.
2. Add lentils, sweet potatoes, kale, vegetable broth, cumin, smoked paprika, salt, and pepper.
3. Bring to a boil, then simmer for 35-40 minutes.
4. Adjust seasoning and serve hot.

Serving Methods:

- Top with a dollop of Greek yogurt.
- Serve with a sprinkle of chopped fresh parsley.

Cauliflower and Turmeric Soup

An anti-inflammatory soup featuring cauliflower and turmeric, providing a delicious blend of flavors with added health benefits for joint support and overall well-being.

Ingredients:

- 1 medium cauliflower, chopped
- 1 onion, chopped
- 3 cloves garlic, minced
- 2 teaspoons ground turmeric
- 8 cups vegetable broth
- 1/2 cup coconut milk
- Salt and pepper to taste

Prep Time: 15 minutes

Cooking Time: 30 minutes

Serving Size: 1 cup

Serving Time: Lunch or Dinner

Nutritional Information (per serving):

- Calories: 160
- Protein: 5g
- Fiber: 6g
- Healthy Fats: 7g

Directions:

1. In a large pot, sauté onion and garlic until softened.
2. Add chopped cauliflower, ground turmeric, vegetable broth, coconut milk, salt, and pepper.
3. Bring to a boil, then simmer for 25-30 minutes.

4. Blend until smooth and serve hot.

Serving Methods:

- Drizzle with extra coconut milk.
- Serve with a sprinkle of ground black pepper.

Artichoke and White Bean Soup

A protein and fiber-packed soup featuring artichokes and white beans, creating a hearty and satisfying option for seniors looking to support their metabolism.

Ingredients: 1 can (14 oz) artichoke hearts, drained and chopped

- 2 cans (15 oz each) cannellini beans, drained and rinsed
- 1 onion, chopped
- 3 cloves garlic, minced
- 8 cups vegetable broth
- 1 teaspoon dried thyme
- 1 teaspoon dried rosemary
- Salt and pepper to taste

Prep Time: 15 minutes

Cooking Time: 30 minutes

Serving Size: 1 cup

Serving Time: Lunch or Dinner

Nutritional Information (per serving):

- Calories: 180
- Protein: 10g
- Fiber: 8g
- Healthy Fats: 2g

Directions:

1. In a large pot, sauté onion and garlic until translucent.
2. Add chopped artichoke hearts, cannellini beans, vegetable broth, thyme, rosemary, salt, and pepper.

3. Bring to a boil, then simmer for 25-30 minutes.
4. Adjust seasoning and serve hot.

Serving Methods:

- Sprinkle with grated Parmesan cheese.
- Serve with a slice of whole-grain bread.

Broccoli and Quinoa Chowder

A wholesome chowder featuring broccoli and quinoa, offering a balance of protein, fiber, and vitamins for a nutritious and comforting meal.

Ingredients: 1 cup quinoa, uncooked

- 4 cups broccoli florets
- 1 onion, finely chopped
- 3 cloves garlic, minced
- 8 cups vegetable broth
- 1 cup almond milk
- 2 tablespoons nutritional yeast
- Salt and pepper to taste

Prep Time: 20 minutes

Cooking Time: 30 minutes

Serving Size: 1 cup

Serving Time: Lunch or Dinner

Nutritional Information (per serving):

- Calories: 210
- Protein: 10g
- Fiber: 8g
- Healthy Fats: 4g

Directions:

1. Rinse quinoa under cold water.
2. In a large pot, sauté onion and garlic until softened.

3. Add quinoa, broccoli, vegetable broth, almond milk, nutritional yeast, salt, and pepper.
4. Bring to a boil, then simmer for 25-30 minutes.
5. Adjust seasoning and serve hot.

Serving Methods:

- Garnish with chopped chives.
- Serve with a side of whole-grain crackers.

Spiced Carrot and Red Lentil Soup

A warming and spiced soup featuring carrots and red lentils, providing a burst of flavor and a robust combination of protein and fiber for metabolic health.

Ingredients:

- 1 cup red lentils, rinsed
- 6 carrots, peeled and chopped
- 1 onion, chopped
- 3 cloves garlic, minced
- 8 cups vegetable broth
- 1 teaspoon ground cumin
- 1/2 teaspoon ground coriander
- 1/4 teaspoon cayenne pepper
- Salt and pepper to taste

Prep Time: 15 minutes

Cooking Time: 30 minutes

Serving Size: 1 cup

Serving Time: Lunch or Dinner

Nutritional Information (per serving):

- Calories: 190
- Protein: 11g
- Fiber: 8g

- Healthy Fats: 1g

Directions:

1. In a large pot, sauté onion and garlic until translucent.
2. Add red lentils, chopped carrots, vegetable broth, cumin, coriander, cayenne pepper, salt, and pepper.
3. Bring to a boil, then simmer for 25-30 minutes.
4. Adjust seasoning and serve hot.

Serving Methods:

- Top with a dollop of Greek yogurt.
- Serve with a sprinkle of fresh cilantro.

Mushroom and Wild Rice Soup

A hearty soup featuring mushrooms and wild rice, offering a delightful texture and a rich umami flavor for a satisfying and nutritious option.

Ingredients:

- 1 cup wild rice, uncooked
- 2 cups mushrooms, sliced
- 1 onion, finely chopped
- 3 cloves garlic, minced
- 8 cups vegetable broth
- 1/2 cup dry white wine (optional)
- 1 teaspoon dried thyme
- 1 teaspoon soy sauce
- Salt and pepper to taste

Prep Time: 20 minutes

Cooking Time: 45 minutes

Serving Size: 1 cup

Serving Time: Lunch or Dinner

Nutritional Information (per serving):

- Calories: 200

- Protein: 7g
- Fiber: 6g
- Healthy Fats: 1g

Directions:

1. Cook wild rice according to package instructions.
2. In a large pot, sauté onion and garlic until softened.
3. Add sliced mushrooms, cooked wild rice, vegetable broth, white wine (if using), thyme, soy sauce, salt, and pepper.
4. Simmer for 35-40 minutes until mushrooms are tender.
5. Adjust seasoning and serve hot.

Serving Methods:

- Garnish with chopped fresh parsley.
- Serve with a slice of crusty whole-grain bread.

Lemon Chickpea and Kale Soup

A refreshing and protein-packed soup featuring chickpeas, kale, and a burst of lemon, providing a light and invigorating option for seniors.

Ingredients:

- 2 cans (15 oz each) chickpeas, drained and rinsed
- 4 cups kale, chopped
- 1 lemon, juiced and zested
- 1 onion, chopped
- 3 cloves garlic, minced
- 8 cups vegetable broth
- 1 teaspoon dried thyme
- 1 teaspoon olive oil
- Salt and pepper to taste

Prep Time: 15 minutes

Cooking Time: 30 minutes

Serving Size: 1 cup

Serving Time: Lunch or Dinner

Nutritional Information (per serving):

- Calories: 180
- Protein: 9g
- Fiber: 8g
- Healthy Fats: 3g

Directions:

1. In a large pot, sauté onion and garlic until translucent.
2. Add chickpeas, chopped kale, vegetable broth, thyme, olive oil, lemon juice, and zest, salt, and pepper.
3. Bring to a boil, then simmer for 25-30 minutes.
4. Adjust seasoning and serve hot.

Serving Methods:

- Drizzle with extra olive oil.
- Serve with a wedge of fresh lemon.

Beet and Quinoa Soup

A vibrant and antioxidant-rich soup featuring beets and quinoa, offering a unique combination of flavors and a boost of essential nutrients for senior health.

Ingredients:

- 2 medium beets, peeled and diced
- 1 cup quinoa, uncooked
- 1 onion, finely chopped
- 3 cloves garlic, minced
- 8 cups vegetable broth
- 1 teaspoon dried dill
- 1/4 cup apple cider vinegar
- Salt and pepper to taste

Prep Time: 20 minutes

Cooking Time: 40 minutes

Serving Size: 1 cup

Serving Time: Lunch or Dinner

Nutritional Information (per serving):

- Calories: 190
- Protein: 7g
- Fiber: 5g
- Healthy Fats: 2g

Directions:

1. Rinse quinoa under cold water.
2. In a large pot, sauté onion and garlic until softened.
3. Add diced beets, quinoa, vegetable broth, dried dill, apple cider vinegar, salt, and pepper.
4. Bring to a boil, then simmer for 35-40 minutes.
5. Adjust seasoning and serve hot.

Serving Methods:

- Garnish with a dollop of Greek yogurt.
- Serve with a sprinkle of fresh parsley.

Black Bean and Corn Soup

A flavorful and protein-rich soup featuring black beans and corn, creating a Tex-Mex-inspired dish with a balance of nutrients and bold taste.

Ingredients:

- 2 cans (15 oz each) black beans, drained and rinsed
- 2 cups corn kernels (fresh or frozen)
- 1 onion, chopped
- 3 cloves garlic, minced
- 1 red bell pepper, diced
- 8 cups vegetable broth
- 1 teaspoon ground cumin

- 1/2 teaspoon chili powder
- Salt and pepper to taste

Prep Time: 15 minutes

Cooking Time: 30 minutes

Serving Size: 1 cup

Serving Time: Lunch or Dinner

Nutritional Information (per serving):

- Calories: 220
- Protein: 11g
- Fiber: 8g
- Healthy Fats: 1g

Directions:

1. In a large pot, sauté onion and garlic until translucent.
2. Add black beans, corn, diced bell pepper, vegetable broth, cumin, chili powder, salt, and pepper.
3. Bring to a boil, then simmer for 25-30 minutes.
4. Adjust seasoning and serve hot.

Serving Methods:

- Top with a spoonful of salsa.
- Serve with a wedge of lime.

Asparagus and Quinoa Soup

A light and detoxifying soup featuring asparagus and quinoa, providing a refreshing option with a blend of vitamins and minerals to support overall health.

Ingredients:

- 1 cup quinoa, uncooked
- 2 cups asparagus, trimmed and chopped
- 1 onion, finely chopped
- 3 cloves garlic, minced

- 8 cups vegetable broth
- 1 lemon, juiced and zested
- 1 tablespoon olive oil
- Salt and pepper to taste

Prep Time: 15 minutes

Cooking Time: 30 minutes

Serving Size: 1 cup

Serving Time: Lunch or Dinner

Nutritional Information (per serving):

- Calories: 180
- Protein: 8g
- Fiber: 6g
- Healthy Fats: 3g

Directions:

1. Rinse quinoa under cold water.
2. In a large pot, sauté onion and garlic until softened.
3. Add chopped asparagus, quinoa, vegetable broth, olive oil, lemon juice, and zest, salt, and pepper.
4. Bring to a boil, then simmer for 25-30 minutes.
5. Adjust seasoning and serve hot.

Serving Methods:

- Drizzle with extra olive oil.
- Serve with a sprinkle of chopped fresh mint.

SEAFOOD RECIPES

Lemon Garlic Baked Salmon

A heart-healthy and flavorful baked salmon dish featuring zesty lemon and garlic for a delicious and quick-to-make option.

Ingredients: 4 salmon fillets

- 2 lemons, sliced
- 4 cloves garlic, minced
- 2 tablespoons olive oil
- 1 teaspoon dried dill
- Salt and pepper to taste

Prep Time: 10 minutes

Cooking Time: 15 minutes

Serving Size: 1 fillet

Serving Time: Lunch or Dinner

Nutritional Information (per serving):

- Calories: 250
- Protein: 25g
- Healthy Fats: 15g
- Omega-3 Fatty Acids: 1.5g

Directions:

1. Preheat the oven to 375°F (190°C).
2. Place salmon fillets on a baking sheet.
3. Drizzle with olive oil, sprinkle minced garlic, dried dill, salt, and pepper.
4. Arrange lemon slices on top.
5. Bake for 15 minutes or until salmon flakes easily with a fork.
6. Serve hot.

Serving Methods:

- Pair with a side of steamed asparagus.

- Serve over a bed of quinoa.

Grilled Shrimp Skewers with Herbs

A light and protein-rich option featuring succulent grilled shrimp seasoned with fresh herbs for a delightful and easy-to-prepare seafood dish.

Ingredients:

- 1 pound large shrimp, peeled and deveined
- 2 tablespoons olive oil
- 2 tablespoons fresh parsley, chopped
- 1 tablespoon fresh dill, chopped
- 1 tablespoon lemon juice
- Salt and pepper to taste

Prep Time: 15 minutes

Cooking Time: 6 minutes

Serving Size: 4 skewers

Serving Time: Lunch or Dinner

Nutritional Information (per serving):

- Calories: 180
- Protein: 20g
- Healthy Fats: 8g

Directions:

1. Preheat the grill to medium-high heat.
2. In a bowl, toss shrimp with olive oil, parsley, dill, lemon juice, salt, and pepper.
3. Thread shrimp onto skewers.
4. Grill for 3 minutes per side or until opaque.
5. Serve hot.

Serving Methods:

- Pair with a side of quinoa salad.

- Serve over a bed of mixed greens.

Baked Cod with Tomato and Olive Tapenad

A Mediterranean-inspired baked cod featuring a vibrant tomato and olive tapenade, providing a burst of flavors and essential nutrients.

Ingredients: 4 cod fillets

- 1 cup cherry tomatoes, halved
- 1/2 cup Kalamata olives, pitted and chopped
- 2 tablespoons capers, drained
- 2 tablespoons fresh basil, chopped
- 1 tablespoon olive oil
- Salt and pepper to taste

Prep Time: 15 minutes

Cooking Time: 20 minutes

Serving Size: 1 fillet

Serving Time: Lunch or Dinner

Nutritional Information (per serving):

- Calories: 220
- Protein: 25g
- Healthy Fats: 9g

Directions:

1. Preheat the oven to 400°F (200°C).
2. Place cod fillets in a baking dish.
3. In a bowl, combine cherry tomatoes, olives, capers, basil, olive oil, salt, and pepper.
4. Spoon the mixture over the cod.
5. Bake for 20 minutes or until fish flakes easily.
6. Serve hot.

Serving Methods:

- Pair with a side of quinoa.

- Serve over a bed of sautéed spinach.

Citrus Glazed Grilled Swordfish

A citrus-infused grilled swordfish dish, providing a unique and refreshing flavor with a good dose of protein and healthy fats.

Ingredients:

- 4 swordfish steaks
- 1/4 cup orange juice
- 2 tablespoons lime juice
- 2 tablespoons honey
- 1 teaspoon fresh thyme, chopped
- Salt and pepper to taste

Prep Time: 15 minutes

Cooking Time: 8 minutes

Serving Size: 1 steak

Serving Time: Lunch or Dinner

Nutritional Information (per serving):

- Calories: 280
- Protein: 30g
- Healthy Fats: 8g

Directions:

1. Preheat the grill to medium-high heat.
2. In a bowl, whisk together orange juice, lime juice, honey, thyme, salt, and pepper.
3. Brush the swordfish steaks with the citrus glaze.
4. Grill for 4 minutes per side or until fish is opaque.
5. Serve hot.

Serving Methods:

- Pair with a side of quinoa and roasted vegetables.
- Serve over a bed of couscous.

Poached Halibut with Herbed Lemon Sauce

A light and poached halibut dish served with a zesty herbed lemon sauce, offering a delicate yet flavorful option for seniors.

Ingredients:

- 4 halibut fillets
- 1/4 cup chicken broth
- 2 tablespoons fresh lemon juice
- 1 tablespoon fresh dill, chopped
- 1 tablespoon fresh parsley, chopped
- 1 teaspoon olive oil
- Salt and pepper to taste

Prep Time: 10 minutes

Cooking Time: 15 minutes

Serving Size: 1 fillet

Serving Time: Lunch or Dinner

Nutritional Information (per serving):

- Calories: 200
- Protein: 28g
- Healthy Fats: 6g

Directions:

1. In a skillet, combine chicken broth, lemon juice, dill, parsley, olive oil, salt, and pepper.
2. Bring to a simmer.
3. Add halibut fillets and poach for 5-7 minutes or until fish is opaque.
4. Serve hot with the herbed lemon sauce.

Serving Methods:

- Pair with a side of quinoa and steamed broccoli.
- Serve over a bed of sautéed spinach.

Garlic Butter Baked Shrimp

A simple and indulgent baked shrimp dish featuring a garlic butter sauce, providing a rich flavor without compromising on nutritional value.

Ingredients:

- 1 pound large shrimp, peeled and deveined
- 4 tablespoons unsalted butter, melted
- 4 cloves garlic, minced
- 2 tablespoons fresh parsley, chopped
- 1 teaspoon lemon zest
- Salt and pepper to taste

Prep Time: 10 minutes

Cooking Time: 12 minutes

Serving Size: 1/2 cup

Serving Time: Lunch or Dinner

Nutritional Information (per serving):

- Calories: 220
- Protein: 22g
- Healthy Fats: 14g

Directions:

1. Preheat the oven to 375°F (190°C).
2. In a bowl, toss shrimp with melted butter, minced garlic, parsley, lemon zest, salt, and pepper.
3. Spread shrimp on a baking sheet.
4. Bake for 10-12 minutes or until shrimp is pink and opaque.
5. Serve hot.

Serving Methods:

- Pair with a side of quinoa and roasted vegetables.
- Serve over a bed of whole-grain pasta.

Asian-Inspired Grilled Tuna Steaks

An Asian-inspired grilled tuna steak marinated in soy, ginger, and sesame, offering a flavorful and protein-packed seafood option.

Ingredients: 4 tuna steaks, 1/4 cup soy sauce (low-sodium)

- 2 tablespoons sesame oil
- 1 tablespoon fresh ginger, grated
- 2 cloves garlic, minced
- 1 tablespoon sesame seeds
- Green onions for garnish

Prep Time: 15 minutes

Marinating Time: 30 minutes

Cooking Time: 6 minutes

Serving Size: 1 steak

Serving Time: Lunch or Dinner

Nutritional Information (per serving):

- Calories: 250
- Protein: 30g
- Healthy Fats: 12g

Directions:

1. In a bowl, whisk together soy sauce, sesame oil, ginger, garlic, and sesame seeds.
2. Marinate tuna steaks for 30 minutes.
3. Preheat the grill to medium-high heat.
4. Grill tuna for 3 minutes per side or until desired doneness.
5. Garnish with chopped green onions.
6. Serve hot.

Serving Methods:

- Pair with a side of brown rice and stir-fried vegetables.
- Serve over a bed of soba noodles.

Mediterranean Baked Haddock

A Mediterranean-inspired baked haddock dish with tomatoes, olives, and herbs, providing a burst of flavors and essential nutrients.

Ingredients:

- 4 haddock fillets
- 1 cup cherry tomatoes, halved
- 1/2 cup Kalamata olives, pitted and sliced
- 2 tablespoons fresh basil, chopped
- 1 tablespoon olive oil
- Salt and pepper to taste

Prep Time: 15 minutes

Cooking Time: 20 minutes

Serving Size: 1 fillet

Serving Time: Lunch or Dinner

Nutritional Information (per serving):

- Calories: 190
- Protein: 24g
- Healthy Fats: 7g

Directions:

1. Preheat the oven to 400°F (200°C).
2. Place haddock fillets in a baking dish.
3. In a bowl, combine cherry tomatoes, olives, basil, olive oil, salt, and pepper.
4. Spoon the mixture over the haddock.
5. Bake for 20 minutes or until fish flakes easily.
6. Serve hot.

Serving Methods:

- Pair with a side of quinoa.
- Serve over a bed of couscous.

Cilantro Lime Grilled Red Snapper

A refreshing and zesty grilled red snapper dish featuring a cilantro lime marinade, offering a burst of flavors and essential nutrients.

Ingredients:

- 4 red snapper fillets
- 1/4 cup fresh cilantro, chopped
- 2 limes, juiced and zested
- 2 tablespoons olive oil
- 1 teaspoon ground cumin
- Salt and pepper to taste

Prep Time: 15 minutes

Marinating Time: 20 minutes

Cooking Time: 6 minutes

Serving Size: 1 fillet

Serving Time: Lunch or Dinner

Nutritional Information (per serving):

- Calories: 230
- Protein: 26g
- Healthy Fats: 10g

Directions:

1. In a bowl, combine cilantro, lime juice, lime zest, olive oil, ground cumin, salt, and pepper.
2. Marinate red snapper fillets for 20 minutes.
3. Preheat the grill to medium-high heat.
4. Grill snapper for 3 minutes per side or until fish is opaque.
5. Serve hot.

Serving Methods:

- Pair with a side of quinoa and avocado salsa.
- Serve over a bed of mixed greens.

Baked Miso Glazed Cod

A flavorful and umami-packed baked cod featuring a miso glaze, providing a unique twist and a boost of protein.

Ingredients:

- 4 cod fillets
- 1/4 cup white miso paste
- 2 tablespoons soy sauce (low-sodium)
- 1 tablespoon rice vinegar
- 1 tablespoon honey
- 1 teaspoon sesame oil
- Sesame seeds for garnish

Prep Time: 15 minutes

Cooking Time: 18 minutes

Serving Size: 1 fillet

Serving Time: Lunch or Dinner

Nutritional Information (per serving):

- Calories: 210
- Protein: 24g
- Healthy Fats: 5g

Directions:

1. Preheat the oven to 400°F (200°C).
2. In a bowl, whisk together miso paste, soy sauce, rice vinegar, honey, and sesame oil.
3. Place cod fillets in a baking dish and brush with the miso glaze.
4. Bake for 18 minutes or until fish flakes easily.
5. Garnish with sesame seeds.
6. Serve hot.

Serving Methods:

- Pair with a side of brown rice and steamed broccoli.
- Serve over a bed of soba noodles.

Herb-Crusted Baked Tilapia

A light and flavorful baked tilapia dish with a herb-infused crust, providing a healthy and quick-to-make option for seniors.

Ingredients: 4 tilapia fillets, 2 tablespoons fresh parsley, chopped

- 1 tablespoon fresh thyme, chopped
- 1 tablespoon olive oil
- 1 tablespoon lemon juice
- Salt and pepper to taste

Prep Time: 10 minutes

Cooking Time: 15 minutes

Serving Size: 1 fillet

Serving Time: Lunch or Dinner

Nutritional Information (per serving):

- Calories: 180
- Protein: 25g
- Healthy Fats: 8g

Directions:

1. Preheat the oven to 375°F (190°C).
2. Mix chopped parsley, thyme, olive oil, lemon juice, salt, and pepper.
3. Coat tilapia fillets with the herb mixture.
4. Bake for 15 minutes or until fish flakes easily.
5. Serve hot.

Serving Methods:

- Pair with a side of quinoa and steamed vegetables.

- Serve over a bed of mixed greens.

Coconut-Curry Shrimp Stir-Fry

A vibrant and exotic shrimp stir-fry with coconut and curry flavors, offering a balance of nutrients and a delightful taste.

Ingredients:

- 1 pound large shrimp, peeled and deveined
- 1 cup broccoli florets
- 1 bell pepper, sliced
- 1 cup snap peas
- 1 can (14 oz) coconut milk
- 2 tablespoons curry powder
- 1 tablespoon coconut oil
- Salt and pepper to taste

Prep Time: 15 minutes

Cooking Time: 10 minutes

Serving Size: 1 cup

Serving Time: Lunch or Dinner

Nutritional Information (per serving):

- Calories: 220
- Protein: 20g
- Healthy Fats: 15g

Directions:

1. In a wok or skillet, heat coconut oil over medium-high heat.
2. Add shrimp, broccoli, bell pepper, and snap peas.
3. Stir-fry for 5-7 minutes until shrimp is pink and vegetables are tender.
4. Pour in coconut milk, add curry powder, salt, and pepper.
5. Simmer for an additional 3 minutes.
6. Serve hot.

Serving Methods:

- Pair with a side of brown rice.
- Serve over cauliflower rice.

Almond-Crusted Cod with Mango Salsa

A crunchy almond-crusted cod paired with a refreshing mango salsa, creating a tropical and nutrient-rich dish for seniors.

Ingredients:

- 4 cod fillets
- 1 cup almonds, finely chopped
- 1 teaspoon paprika
- 1/2 teaspoon garlic powder
- 1 mango, diced
- 1/2 red onion, finely chopped
- 1 jalapeño, seeded and minced
- 2 tablespoons fresh cilantro, chopped
- 1 lime, juiced
- Salt and pepper to taste

Prep Time: 20 minutes

Cooking Time: 12 minutes

Serving Size: 1 fillet

Serving Time: Lunch or Dinner

Nutritional Information (per serving):

- Calories: 250
- Protein: 28g
- Healthy Fats: 14g

Directions:

1. Preheat the oven to 400°F (200°C).
2. Mix chopped almonds, paprika, garlic powder, salt, and pepper.
3. Coat cod fillets with the almond mixture.

4. Bake for 12 minutes or until fish flakes easily.
5. In a bowl, combine mango, red onion, jalapeño, cilantro, lime juice, salt, and pepper for salsa.
6. Serve cod topped with mango salsa.

Serving Methods:

- Pair with a side of quinoa.
- Serve over a bed of arugula.

Teriyaki Glazed Salmon

A savory and sweet teriyaki-glazed salmon, providing omega-3 fatty acids and a burst of Asian-inspired flavors.

Ingredients: 4 salmon fillets

- 1/4 cup low-sodium soy sauce
- 2 tablespoons honey
- 1 tablespoon rice vinegar
- 1 teaspoon sesame oil
- 1 tablespoon ginger, grated
- 2 cloves garlic, minced
- Green onions for garnish

Prep Time: 15 minutes

Cooking Time: 10 minutes

Serving Size: 1 fillet

Serving Time: Lunch or Dinner

Nutritional Information (per serving):

- Calories: 280
- Protein: 26g
- Healthy Fats: 15g

Directions:

1. In a bowl, whisk together soy sauce, honey, rice vinegar, sesame oil, ginger, and garlic.

2. Marinate salmon fillets for 10 minutes.
3. Preheat the grill or skillet to medium-high heat.
4. Grill salmon for 5 minutes per side or until fish is opaque.
5. Garnish with chopped green onions.
6. Serve hot.

Serving Methods:

- Pair with a side of brown rice and steamed broccoli.
- Serve over a bed of soba noodles.

Lemon Herb Baked Scallops

Delicate and flavorful baked scallops with a zesty lemon-herb seasoning, offering a light and protein-packed seafood option.

Ingredients: 1 pound scallops

- 2 tablespoons olive oil
- 1 lemon, juiced and zested
- 2 tablespoons fresh parsley, chopped
- 1 tablespoon fresh thyme, chopped
- Salt and pepper to taste

Prep Time: 10 minutes

Cooking Time: 12 minutes

Serving Size: 1/2 cup

Serving Time: Lunch or Dinner

Nutritional Information (per serving):

- Calories: 160
- Protein: 20g
- Healthy Fats: 8g

Directions:

1. Preheat the oven to 400°F (200°C).
2. In a bowl, toss scallops with olive oil, lemon juice, lemon zest, parsley, thyme, salt, and pepper.

3. Arrange scallops on a baking sheet.
4. Bake for 12 minutes or until scallops are opaque.
5. Serve hot.

Serving Methods:

- Pair with a side of quinoa and roasted vegetables.
- Serve over a bed of spinach.

Pesto Grilled Trout

An herbaceous and grilled trout dish featuring a vibrant pesto marinade, providing a delicious and nutrient-rich option.

Ingredients: 4 trout fillets

- 1 cup fresh basil leaves
- 1/2 cup pine nuts
- 1/2 cup Parmesan cheese, grated
- 2 cloves garlic
- 1/2 cup olive oil
- Salt and pepper to taste

Prep Time: 15 minutes

Marinating Time: 30 minutes

Cooking Time: 8 minutes

Serving Size: 1 fillet

Serving Time: Lunch or Dinner

Nutritional Information (per serving):

- Calories: 260
- Protein: 22g
- Healthy Fats: 18g

Directions:

1. In a blender, combine basil, pine nuts, Parmesan, garlic, salt, and pepper.

2. While blending, slowly add olive oil until a pesto consistency is achieved.
3. Marinate trout fillets in pesto for 30 minutes.
4. Preheat the grill to medium-high heat.
5. Grill trout for 4 minutes per side or until fish is opaque.
6. Serve hot.

Serving Methods:

- Pair with a side of quinoa and sautéed kale.
- Serve over a bed of couscous.

Baked Crab-Stuffed Avocado

A unique and indulgent baked dish featuring crab-stuffed avocados, offering a combination of healthy fats and protein.

Ingredients: 2 avocados, halved and pitted

- 1 cup lump crab meat
- 1/4 cup mayonnaise (light)
- 1 tablespoon Dijon mustard
- 1 tablespoon fresh lemon juice
- 2 tablespoons fresh chives, chopped
- Salt and pepper to taste

Prep Time: 15 minutes

Cooking Time: 15 minutes

Serving Size: 1 half avocado

Serving Time: Lunch or Dinner

Nutritional Information (per serving):

- Calories: 220
- Protein: 15g
- Healthy Fats: 18g

Directions:

1. Preheat the oven to 375°F (190°C).

2. In a bowl, mix crab meat, mayonnaise, Dijon mustard, lemon juice, chives, salt, and pepper.
3. Spoon crab mixture into avocado halves.
4. Place avocados on a baking sheet.
5. Bake for 15 minutes or until crab mixture is heated through.
6. Serve hot.

Serving Methods:

- Pair with a side of mixed greens.
- Serve over a bed of arugula.

Cumin-Spiced Grilled Mahi-Mahi

A spice-infused grilled mahi-mahi with cumin, offering a bold and protein-rich option for seniors.

Ingredients: 4 mahi-mahi fillets

- 1 tablespoon ground cumin
- 1 teaspoon smoked paprika
- 1 teaspoon garlic powder
- 1 tablespoon olive oil
- Lime wedges for garnish
- Salt and pepper to taste

Prep Time: 10 minutes

Cooking Time: 8 minutes

Serving Size: 1 fillet

Serving Time: Lunch or Dinner

Nutritional Information (per serving):

- Calories: 240
- Protein: 28g
- Healthy Fats: 10g

Directions:

1. Preheat the grill to medium-high heat.

2. In a bowl, mix cumin, paprika, garlic powder, olive oil, salt, and pepper.
3. Coat mahi-mahi fillets with the spice mixture.
4. Grill for 4 minutes per side or until fish is opaque.
5. Garnish with lime wedges.
6. Serve hot.

Serving Methods:

- Pair with a side of quinoa and black beans.
- Serve over a bed of brown rice.

Lemon Dill Baked Oysters

A sophisticated yet easy-to-make baked oyster dish with a lemon dill drizzle, providing a unique seafood option for seniors.

Ingredients:

- 12 fresh oysters, shucked
- 2 tablespoons unsalted butter, melted
- 1 tablespoon fresh dill, chopped
- 1 lemon, juiced and zested
- Salt and pepper to taste

Prep Time: 15 minutes

Cooking Time: 10 minutes

Serving Size: 6 oysters

Serving Time: Lunch or Dinner

Nutritional Information (per serving):

- Calories: 180
- Protein: 12g
- Healthy Fats: 14g

Directions:

1. Preheat the oven to 425°F (220°C).
2. Place shucked oysters on a baking sheet.

3. In a bowl, mix melted butter, dill, lemon juice, lemon zest, salt, and pepper.
4. Drizzle the mixture over the oysters.
5. Bake for 10 minutes or until edges are golden.
6. Serve hot.

Serving Methods:

- Pair with a side of crusty whole-grain bread.
- Serve over a bed of arugula.

Spicy Garlic Grilled Squid

A bold and spicy grilled squid dish with garlic, offering a unique texture and a flavorful kick.

Ingredients:

- 1 pound cleaned squid tubes and tentacles
- 2 tablespoons olive oil
- 2 cloves garlic, minced
- 1 teaspoon red pepper flakes
- 1 tablespoon fresh parsley, chopped
- 1 lemon, cut into wedges
- Salt and pepper to taste

Prep Time: 20 minutes

Cooking Time: 6 minutes

Serving Size: 1 cup

Serving Time: Lunch or Dinner

Nutritional Information (per serving):

- Calories: 160
- Protein: 20g
- Healthy Fats: 8g

Directions:

1. Preheat the grill to medium-high heat.

2. In a bowl, toss cleaned squid with olive oil, minced garlic, red pepper flakes, salt, and pepper.
3. Grill squid for 2-3 minutes per side or until opaque.
4. Sprinkle with fresh parsley and serve with lemon wedges.
5. Serve hot.

Serving Methods:

- Pair with a side of quinoa and grilled vegetables.
- Serve over a bed of mixed greens.

28 DAY MEAL PLAN

Day 1:

- *Breakfast:* Herb-Crusted Baked Tilapia with Mixed Greens
- *Lunch:* Coconut-Curry Shrimp Stir-Fry with Brown Rice
- *Dinner:* Almond-Crusted Cod with Mango Salsa over Quinoa

Day 2:

- *Breakfast:* Lemon Herb Baked Scallops with Steamed Broccoli
- *Lunch:* Teriyaki Glazed Salmon with Soba Noodles
- *Dinner:* Pesto Grilled Trout with Couscous and Sautéed Kale

Day 3:

- *Breakfast:* Baked Crab-Stuffed Avocado with Mixed Greens
- *Lunch:* Cumin-Spiced Grilled Mahi-Mahi with Quinoa and Black Beans
- *Dinner:* Lemon Dill Baked Oysters with Crusty Whole-Grain Bread

Day 4:

- *Breakfast:* Spicy Garlic Grilled Squid with Quinoa and Grilled Vegetables
- *Lunch:* Grilled Shrimp Skewers with Herbs over Brown Rice
- *Dinner:* Mediterranean Baked Haddock with Couscous

Day 5:

- *Breakfast:* Citrus Glazed Grilled Swordfish with a Side of Mixed Berries
- *Lunch:* Baked Miso Glazed Cod with Brown Rice and Steamed Broccoli
- *Dinner:* Asian-Inspired Grilled Tuna Steaks with Stir-Fried Vegetables

Day 6:

- *Breakfast:* Cilantro Lime Grilled Red Snapper with Quinoa and Avocado Salsa
- *Lunch:* Baked Crab-Stuffed Avocado with Arugula Salad
- *Dinner:* Lemon Garlic Baked Salmon with Asparagus

Day 7:

- *Breakfast:* Pesto Grilled Trout with a Side of Fresh Fruit
- *Lunch:* Teriyaki Glazed Salmon over a Bed of Spinach
- *Dinner:* Almond-Crusted Cod with Mango Salsa over Mixed Greens

Day 8:

- *Breakfast:* Coconut-Curry Shrimp Stir-Fry with Cauliflower Rice
- *Lunch:* Mediterranean Baked Haddock with Quinoa
- *Dinner:* Spicy Garlic Grilled Squid with Mixed Greens

Day 9:

- *Breakfast:* Baked Miso Glazed Cod with a Side of Fresh Berries
- *Lunch:* Lemon Dill Baked Oysters over a Bed of Arugula
- *Dinner:* Asian-Inspired Grilled Tuna Steaks with Stir-Fried Vegetables

Day 10:

- *Breakfast:* Herb-Crusted Baked Tilapia with Quinoa and Steamed Broccoli
- *Lunch:* Cumin-Spiced Grilled Mahi-Mahi with Brown Rice and Black Beans
- *Dinner:* Pesto Grilled Trout with Couscous and Sautéed Kale

Day 11:

- *Breakfast:* Lemon Herb Baked Scallops with Mixed Berries
- *Lunch:* Teriyaki Glazed Salmon with Soba Noodles
- *Dinner:* Almond-Crusted Cod with Mango Salsa over Mixed Greens

Day 12:

- *Breakfast:* Baked Crab-Stuffed Avocado with a Side of Fresh Fruit
- *Lunch:* Grilled Shrimp Skewers with Herbs over Brown Rice
- *Dinner:* Mediterranean Baked Haddock with Quinoa

Day 13:

- *Breakfast:* Citrus Glazed Grilled Swordfish with Steamed Asparagus
- *Lunch:* Baked Miso Glazed Cod with Brown Rice and Steamed Broccoli
- *Dinner:* Asian-Inspired Grilled Tuna Steaks with Stir-Fried Vegetables

Day 14:

- *Breakfast:* Cilantro Lime Grilled Red Snapper with Quinoa and Avocado Salsa
- *Lunch:* Baked Crab-Stuffed Avocado with Arugula Salad
- *Dinner:* Lemon Garlic Baked Salmon with Roasted Sweet Potatoes

Day 15:

- *Breakfast:* Coconut-Curry Shrimp Stir-Fry with Cauliflower Rice
- *Lunch:* Mediterranean Baked Haddock with Quinoa

- *Dinner:* Spicy Garlic Grilled Squid with Mixed Greens

Day 16:

- *Breakfast:* Baked Miso Glazed Cod with a Side of Fresh Berries
- *Lunch:* Lemon Dill Baked Oysters over a Bed of Arugula
- *Dinner:* Asian-Inspired Grilled Tuna Steaks with Stir-Fried Vegetables

Day 17:

- *Breakfast:* Herb-Crusted Baked Tilapia with Quinoa and Steamed Broccoli
- *Lunch:* Cumin-Spiced Grilled Mahi-Mahi with Brown Rice and Black Beans
- *Dinner:* Pesto Grilled Trout with Couscous and Sautéed Kale

Day 18:

- *Breakfast:* Lemon Herb Baked Scallops with Mixed Berries
- *Lunch:* Teriyaki Glazed Salmon with Soba Noodles
- *Dinner:* Almond-Crusted Cod with Mango Salsa over Mixed Greens

Day 19:

- *Breakfast:* Baked Crab-Stuffed Avocado with a Side of Fresh Fruit
- *Lunch:* Grilled Shrimp Skewers with Herbs over Brown Rice
- *Dinner:* Mediterranean Baked Haddock with Quinoa

Day 20:

- *Breakfast:* Citrus Glazed Grilled Swordfish with Steamed Asparagus
- *Lunch:* Baked Miso Glazed Cod with Brown Rice and Steamed Broccoli

- *Dinner:* Asian-Inspired Grilled Tuna Steaks with Stir-Fried Vegetables

Day 21:

- *Breakfast:* Cilantro Lime Grilled Red Snapper with Quinoa and Avocado Salsa

- *Lunch:* Baked Crab-Stuffed Avocado with Arugula Salad

- *Dinner:* Lemon Garlic Baked Salmon with Roasted Sweet Potatoes

Day 22:

- *Breakfast:* Herb-Crusted Baked Tilapia with Mixed Greens

- *Lunch:* Coconut-Curry Shrimp Stir-Fry with Brown Rice

- *Dinner:* Almond-Crusted Cod with Mango Salsa over Quinoa

Day 23:

- *Breakfast:* Lemon Herb Baked Scallops with Steamed Broccoli

- *Lunch:* Teriyaki Glazed Salmon with Soba Noodles

- *Dinner:* Pesto Grilled Trout with Couscous and Sautéed Kale

Day 24:

- *Breakfast:* Baked Crab-Stuffed Avocado with Mixed Greens

- *Lunch:* Cumin-Spiced Grilled Mahi-Mahi with Quinoa and Black Beans

- *Dinner:* Lemon Dill Baked Oysters with Crusty Whole-Grain Bread

Day 25:

- *Breakfast:* Spicy Garlic Grilled Squid with Quinoa and Grilled Vegetables

- *Lunch:* Grilled Shrimp Skewers with Herbs over Brown Rice

- *Dinner:* Mediterranean Baked Haddock with Couscous

Day 26:

- *Breakfast:* Citrus Glazed Grilled Swordfish with a Side of Mixed Berries

- *Lunch: Baked* Miso Glazed Cod with Brown Rice and Steamed Broccoli

- *Dinner:* Asian-Inspired Grilled Tuna Steaks with Stir-Fried Vegetables

Day 27:

- *Breakfast:* Cilantro Lime Grilled Red Snapper with Quinoa and Avocado Salsa

- *Lunch:* Baked Crab-Stuffed Avocado with Arugula Salad

- **Dinner:** Lemon Garlic Baked Salmon with Asparagus

Day 28:

- *Breakfast:* Pesto Grilled Trout with a Side of Fresh Fruit

- *Lunch:* Teriyaki Glazed Salmon over a Bed of Spinach

- *Dinner:* Almond-Crusted Cod with Mango Salsa over Mixed Greens

CONCLUSION

The "Metabolic Reset Cookbook for Seniors" is not just a collection of recipes but a thoughtful guide tailored to address the unique nutritional needs of seniors aiming for a metabolic reset. This cookbook is a comprehensive resource that delves into various aspects, providing a holistic approach to enhance metabolic health in seniors.

The purpose of the cookbook is to serve as a practical tool, offering a diverse array of recipes specifically curated to support metabolic reset. It goes beyond being a mere compilation of dishes, emphasizing the importance of nutrition and lifestyle choices in promoting overall well-being among seniors.

The understanding of metabolism in seniors is explored in depth, shedding light on how metabolic processes evolve with age. This knowledge forms the foundation for the cookbook, ensuring that the recipes are not only delicious but also strategically crafted to align with the changing metabolic dynamics in seniors.

The cookbook systematically addresses the changes in metabolism that occur with age, acknowledging the unique challenges seniors face. By recognizing and understanding these changes, the cookbook empowers seniors to make informed dietary choices that contribute to a healthier and more balanced lifestyle.

Common metabolic challenges for seniors are identified and addressed, providing practical insights and solutions. From incorporating physical activity to stress management and sleep, the cookbook extends its focus beyond the kitchen, recognizing the interconnected nature of lifestyle factors influencing metabolic health.

Vitamins and minerals are highlighted for their crucial role in supporting seniors' health. The cookbook emphasizes the importance of a nutrient-rich diet, offering recipes that not only tantalize the taste buds but also provide essential vitamins and minerals vital for metabolic function.

Hydration, often overlooked, is given due consideration. The cookbook offers professional advice on maintaining optimal hydration, recognizing its impact on metabolic health. Practical tips are provided to ensure seniors can easily incorporate effective hydration practices into their daily routines.

The heart of the cookbook lies in its meticulously curated recipes. From breakfast to dinner, and even side dishes, salads, soups, and seafood, each recipe is not just a culinary delight but a carefully crafted combination of ingredients aimed at supporting metabolic health in seniors. Detailed nutritional information and serving suggestions empower seniors to make choices that align with their individual dietary preferences and requirements.

In crafting a 28-day meal plan, the cookbook takes a step further, providing a structured guide for seniors to follow. This meal plan is a testament to the cookbook's commitment to ensuring that the journey to metabolic reset is not only health-conscious but also flavourful and enjoyable.

Made in United States
Orlando, FL
26 May 2025

61604105R00108